Trigeminal Neuralgia

Editors

JOHN Y.K. LEE
MICHAEL LIM

NEUROSURGERY
CLINICS OF NORTH AMERICA

www.neurosurgery.theclinics.com

Consulting Editors

RUSSELL LONSER
DANIEL K. RESNICK

July 2016 • Volume 27 • Number 3

ELSEVIER

1600 John F. Kennedy Boulevard • Suite 1800 • Philadelphia, Pennsylvania, 19103-2899

http://www.theclinics.com

NEUROSURGERY CLINICS OF NORTH AMERICA Volume 27, Number 3
July 2016 ISSN 1042-3680, ISBN-13: 978-0-323-44849-9

Editor: Jennifer Flynn-Briggs
Developmental Editor: Colleen Viola

Neurosurgery Clinics of North America (ISSN 1042-3680) is published quarterly by Elsevier Inc., 360 Park Avenue South, New York, NY 10010-1710. Months of issue are January, April, July, and October. Business and Editorial Offices: 1600 John F. Kennedy Blvd., Suite 1800, Philadelphia, PA 19103-2899. Customer Service Office: 11830 Westline Industrial Drive, St. Louis, MO 63146. Periodicals postage paid at New York, NY, and additional mailing offices. Subscription prices are $385.00 per year (US individuals), $639.00 per year (US institutions), $415.00 per year (Canadian individuals), $794.00 per year (Canadian institutions), $495.00 per year (international individuals), $794.00 per year (international institutions), $100.00 per year (US students), and $255.00 per year (international and Canadian students). International air speed delivery is included in all *Clinics* subscription prices. All prices are subject to change without notice. **POSTMASTER:** Send address changes to *Neurosurgery Clinics of North America*, Elsevier Periodicals Customer Service, 11830 Westline Industrial Drive, St. Louis, MO 63146. **Customer Service: 1-800-654-2452 (US and Canada). From outside the US and Canada, call: 1-314-453-7041. Fax: 1-314-453-5170. E-mail: JournalsCustomerService-usa@elsevier.com (for print support) and journalsonlinesupport-usa@elsevier.com (for online support).**

Reprints. For copies of 100 or more, of articles in this publication, please contact the Commercial Reprints Department, Elsevier Inc., 360 Park Avenue South, New York, NY 10010-1710. Tel. 212-633-3874; Fax: 212-633-3820; E-mail: reprints@elsevier.com.

Neurosurgery Clinics of North America is covered in *MEDLINE/PubMed (Index Medicus), EMBASE/Excerpta Medica, and Current Contents/Clinical Medicine (CC/CM).*

Contributors

CONSULTING EDITORS

RUSSELL LONSER, MD
Professor and Chair, Department of Neurological Surgery, The Ohio State University Wexner Medical Center, Columbus, Ohio

DANIEL K. RESNICK, MD, MS
Professor and Vice Chairman; Program Director, Department of Neurosurgery, University of Wisconsin School of Medicine and Public Health, Madison, Wisconsin

EDITORS

JOHN Y.K. LEE, MD, MSCE
Associate Professor, Department of Neurosurgery, Pennsylvania Hospital, Perelman School of Medicine at the University of Pennsylvania, Philadelphia, Pennsylvania

MICHAEL LIM, MD
Associate Professor of Neurosurgery, Oncology, Radiation Oncology, and Institute of NanoBiotechnology; Director of the Brain Tumor Immunotherapy Program; Director of the Metastatic Brain Tumor Center, Johns Hopkins University School of Medicine, Baltimore, Maryland

AUTHORS

NAFI AYGUN, MD
Associate Professor, Division of Neuroradiology, The Russel H. Morgan Department of Radiology and Radiologic Science, The Johns Hopkins Hospital, Baltimore, Maryland

MATTHEW T. BENDER, MD
Department of Neurosurgery, Johns Hopkins University School of Medicine, Baltimore, Maryland

CHETAN BETTEGOWDA, MD, PhD
Department of Neurosurgery, Johns Hopkins University School of Medicine, Baltimore, Maryland

ARI M. BLITZ, MD
Director of Skull Base Imaging and Assistant Professor; Division of Neuroradiology, The Russel H. Morgan Department of Radiology and Radiologic Science, The Johns Hopkins Hospital, Baltimore, Maryland

FRANCO DEMONTE, MD
Professor, Department of Neurosurgery, The University of Texas M.D. Anderson Cancer Center, Houston, Texas

DOUGLAS KONDZIOLKA, MD, MSc, FRCSC, FACS
Professor, Vice-Chair, Clinical Research, Department of Neurosurgery, Director, Center for Advanced Radiosurgery, NYU Langone Medical Center, New York, New York

SHIVANAND P. LAD, MD, PhD
Assistant professor, Department of Neurosurgery, Duke University Medical Center, Durham, North Carolina

JOHN Y.K. LEE, MD, MSCE
Associate Professor, Department of Neurosurgery, Pennsylvania Hospital, Perelman School of Medicine at the University of Pennsylvania, Philadelphia, Pennsylvania

JAMES K. LIU, MD, FACS, FAANS
Director, Center for Skull Base and Pituitary Surgery, Associate Professor of Neurological Surgery, Departments of Neurological Surgery and Otolaryngology-Head and Neck Surgery, Neurological Institute of New Jersey, Rutgers University – New Jersey Medical School, Newark, New Jersey

BENJAMIN NORTHCUTT, MD
Clinical Post-doctoral Fellow, Division of Neuroradiology, The Russel H. Morgan Department of Radiology and Radiologic Science, The Johns Hopkins Hospital, Baltimore, Maryland

SMRUTI K. PATEL, MD
Resident in Neurological Surgery, Department of Neurological Surgery, University of Cincinnati Medical Center, University of Cincinnati College of Medicine, Cincinnati, Ohio

JACK PHAN, MD, PhD
Assistant Professor, Department of Radiation Oncology, The University of Texas M.D. Anderson Cancer Center, Houston, Texas

MATTHEW PIAZZA, MD
Resident Neurosurgeon, Department of Neurosurgery, Hospital of the University of Pennsylvania, Perelman School of Medicine at the University of Pennsylvania, Philadelphia, Pennsylvania

SHERVIN RAHIMPOUR, MD
Resident, Director of NeuroInnovations Program, Department of Neurosurgery, Duke University Medical Center, Durham, North Carolina

SHAAN M. RAZA, MD
Assistant Professor, Department of Neurosurgery, The University of Texas M.D. Anderson Cancer Center, Houston, Texas

GADDUM DUEMANI REDDY, MD, PhD
Department of Neurosurgery, The University of Texas M.D. Anderson Cancer Center, Houston, Texas

CLARE RELTON, PhD
Senior Research Fellow, School for Health and related Research, University of Sheffield, Sheffield, United Kingdom

DANIEL P. SEEBURG, MD, PhD
Clinical Post-doctoral Fellow, Division of Neuroradiology, The Russel H. Morgan Department of Radiology and Radiologic Science, The Johns Hopkins Hospital, Baltimore, Maryland

KATHRYN WAGNER, MD
Department of Neurosurgery, The University of Texas M.D. Anderson Cancer Center, Houston, Texas

AMPARO WOLF, MD, PhD
Department of Neurosurgery, NYU Langone Medical Center, New York, New York

JOANNA M. ZAKRZEWSKA, MD
Consultant/Honorary Professor, Division of Diagnostic, Surgical and Medical Sciences, Eastman Dental Hospital, UCLH NHS Foundation Trust, London, United Kingdom

Contents

NEUROSURGERY CLINICS OF NORTH AMERICA

FORTHCOMING ISSUES

October 2016
Traumatic Brain Injury
Daniel Hirt, Paul Vespa, and Geoffrey Manley, *Editors*

January 2017
Adult and Pediatric Spine Trauma
Douglas L. Brockmeyer and Andrew T. Dailey, *Editors*

April 2017
Subdural Hematomas
E. Sander Connolly Jr and Guy M. McKhann II, *Editors*

July 2017
Complications in Neurosurgery
Russell Lonser and Daniel K. Resnick, *Editors*

October 2017
Intraoperative Imaging
J. Bradley Elder and Ganesh Rao, *Editors*

RECENT ISSUES

April 2016
Memingiomas
Gabriel Zada and Randy L. Jensen, *Editors*

January 2016
Epilepsy
Kareem A. Zaghloul and Edward F. Chang, *Editors*

October 2015
Chiari Malformation
Jeffrey Leonard and David Limbrick, *Editors*

July 2015
Endoscopic Endonasal Skull Base Surgery
Daniel M. Prevedello, *Editor*

RELATED INTEREST

Dental Clinics of North America, April 2016 (Vol. 60, Issue 2)
Clinical Pharmacology for Dentists
Harry Dym, *Editor*

Preface

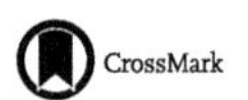

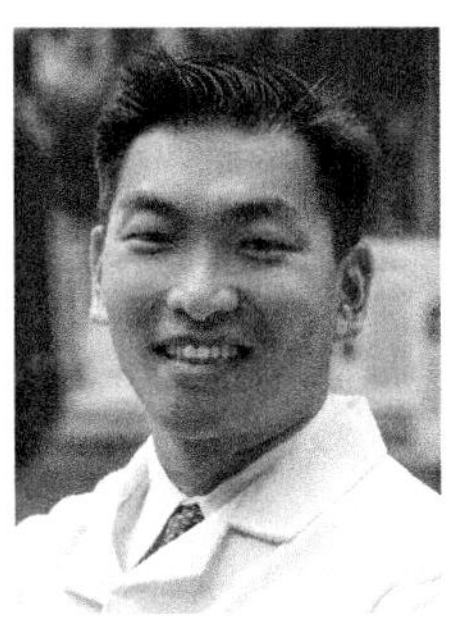

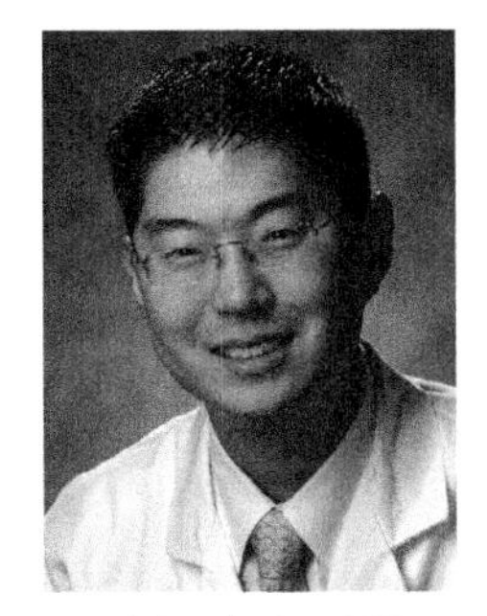

John Y.K. Lee, MD, MSCE Michael Lim, MD
Editors

Trigeminal neuralgia is one of the most common causes of facial pain and can negatively affect a patient's quality of life. Trigeminal neuralgia has always been of significant interest to neurosurgeons at least since 1820 when Charles Bell first described the anatomy of the trigeminal nerve and separated it from the anatomy and function of the facial nerve. Once the anatomy was established, enterprising surgeons created a variety of techniques to relieve the suffering of their patients. In this issue of *Neurosurgery Clinics of North America*, we provide the reader with an overview of the history as it is impossible to advance the field without appreciation of the past. Furthermore, we critically analyze the current state of current surgical techniques (percutaneous rhizotomy, Gamma Knife stereotactic radiosurgery, microvascular decompression, and even fully endoscopic microvascular decompression). In addition, we look to the future of designing new approaches for the treatment of trigeminal neuralgia by examining the current methods of measuring facial pain and issues for future clinical trials. Finally, we discuss the current state of surgical treatments for atypical facial pain. In this issue, we hope to provide a framework to advance the field.

John Y.K. Lee, MD, MSCE
Department of Neurological Surgery
University of Pennsylvania
235 South Eighth Street
Philadelphia, PA 19106, USA

Michael Lim, MD
Institute of NanoBiotechnology
Johns Hopkins University
School of Medicine
Johns Hopkins Hospital
Neurosurgery-Phipps 123
600 North Wolfe Street
Baltimore, MD 21287, USA

E-mail addresses:
leejohn@uphs.upenn.edu (J.Y.K. Lee)
mlim3@jhmi.edu (M. Lim)

Neurosurg Clin N Am 27 (2016) ix
http://dx.doi.org/10.1016/j.nec.2016.05.001
1042-3680/16/$ – see front matter

Overview and History of Trigeminal Neuralgia

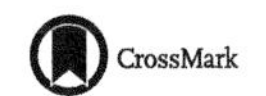

Smruti K. Patel, MD[a], James K. Liu, MD[b,c,*]

KEYWORDS

- Trigeminal neuralgia • Tic douloureux • Percutaneous rhizotomy • Radiofrequency ablation
- Microvascular decompression • Walter Dandy • Peter Jannetta

KEY POINTS

- Although the earliest descriptions of trigeminal neuralgia as a clinical entity date back as early as the 1600s, the term *tic douloureux* was coined nearly a century after in 1756, by Nicholas Andre.
- Ablative techniques included percutaneous ablation with radiofrequency lesioning, glycerol chemoneurolysis, balloon microcompression, and stereotactic radiosurgery.
- Although Dandy initially observed neurovascular compression during his operation of partial trigeminal neurectomy, it was Jannetta who introduced the operating microscope to confirm these findings culminating in the microvascular decompression procedure.

INTRODUCTION

A horrid affliction in its full fury, trigeminal neuralgia (TN), also known as *tic douloureux*, has been a major neurosurgical concern since neurosurgery first emerged as a distinct surgical specialty in the early 20th century.[1] In its classic form, TN results in episodes of intense, lancinating facial pain followed by a period of relief. However, even during these periods of relief, patients often live in fear and anticipation of the next episode. The earliest descriptions of TN as a clinical entity date back to the 1600s provided by prominent physicians at the time including Drs Johannes Michael Fehr and Elias Schmidt, secretaries of the Imperial Leopoldina Academy of the Natural Sciences, and famous philosopher John Locke.[2] However, the term *tic douloureux* was not coined until nearly a century after in 1756, by Nicholas Andre (**Fig. 1**, left) who believed that the condition stemmed from a nerve in distress and classified it as a convulsive disorder.[1] He conceptualized the disease in terms of convulsions and used the term *tic douloureux* to imply contortions and grimaces accompanied by violent and unbearable pain. In 1773, an English physician, Dr. John Fothergill (see **Fig. 1**, right) presented his experience with 14 patient encounters and deemed the cause to be related to cancer rather than a convulsive disorder, thus coining the term, *Fothergill's disease*. In his remarkable and accurate description, he stated, "The affection seems to be peculiar to persons advancing in years, and to women more than to men...The pain comes suddenly and is excruciating; it lasts but a short time, perhaps a

Disclosures: The authors have no financial disclosures.

[a] Department of Neurological Surgery, University of Cincinnati Medical Center, University of Cincinnati College of Medicine, PO Box 670515, Cincinnati, OH 45267-0515, USA; [b] Department of Neurological Surgery, Center for Skull Base and Pituitary Surgery, Neurological Institute of New Jersey, Rutgers University – New Jersey Medical School, 90 Bergen Street, Suite # 8100, Newark, NJ 07103, USA; [c] Department of Otolaryngology-Head and Neck Surgery, Center for Skull Base and Pituitary Surgery, Neurological Institute of New Jersey, Rutgers University – New Jersey Medical School, 90 Bergen Street, Suite # 8100, Newark, NJ 07103, USA
* Corresponding author. Department of Otolaryngology-Head and Neck Surgery, Center for Skull Base and Pituitary Surgery, Neurological Institute of New Jersey, Rutgers University – New Jersey Medical School, 90 Bergen Street, Suite # 8100, Newark, NJ 07103.
E-mail address: james.liu.md@rutgers.edu

Neurosurg Clin N Am 27 (2016) 265–276
http://dx.doi.org/10.1016/j.nec.2016.02.002
1042-3680/16/$ – see front matter

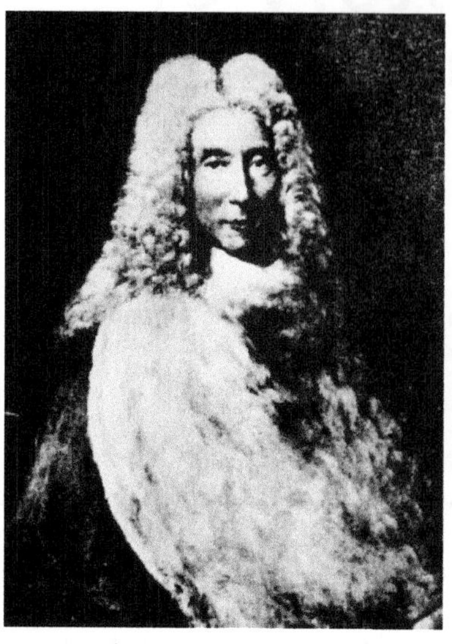
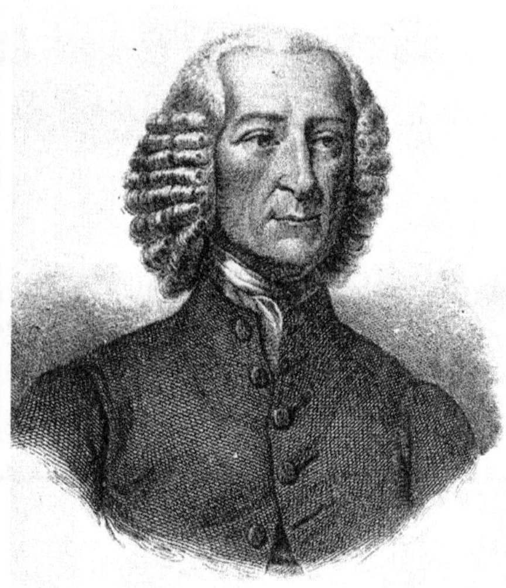

Fig. 1. (*Left*) portrait of Nicolas Andre. (*Right*) portrait of John Fothergill. ([*Left*] *From* Legrand N. Les Collections de la Faculte de Medecine de Paris. Paris: Masson; 1911; and *Courtesy of* the Wellcome Institute Library, London, United Kingdom; and [*Right*] *Reprinted from* Stookey B, Ransohoff J. Trigeminal neuralgia: its history and treatment. Springfield (IL): Charles C Thomas; 1959.)

quarter or half a minute, and then goes off; it returns at irregular intervals, sometimes in half an hour, sometimes there are two or three repetitions in a few minutes...Eating will bring it on some persons. Talking, or the least motion of the muscles of the face affects others; the gentlest touch of a handkerchief will sometimes bring on the pain, whilst a strong pressure on the part has no effect."[3]

Although the clinical description of this condition had been clarified by the end of the 18th century, it was not until the 1820s that Charles Bell localized this pain syndrome to the trigeminal nerve; thus, the condition was ultimately referred to as *trigeminal neuralgia*.[1] Although the cause of TN remained elusive for a long time, a common denominator in most cases was segmental demyelination at the root entry zone of the trigeminal nerve. Some of the recognized causes included vascular compression of the nerve, a compressive mass lesion, postinfectious multiple sclerosis, trigeminal deafferentation, and atypical facial pain that may be related to a somatoform pain disorder. Traditionally, medical therapy is the initial treatment of choice. If the condition becomes medically refractory, various surgical options are described and are available, some with better success rates than others.

Evolution of Therapies for Trigeminal Neuralgia

Medical management

Early medical treatments for the treatment of TN in the 18th and 19th centuries included such compounds as quinine derived from Peruvian bark,[3] mercury, opium, arsenic,[4] and powder of gelsenium.[2] Trichloroethylene and stilbamidine became popular choices for the treatment of facial pain in the early 20th century; however, their side-effect profile precluded them from becoming lasting options.[2,5] The use of antiepileptic medications was first described in 1942 by Bergouignan with the introduction of sodium diphenylhydantoin.[6] By the 1960s, phenytoin and, subsequently, carbamazepine were largely used as the treatments of choice as medical therapies for TN. Several other antiepileptic medications have been introduced to the treatment paradigm including lamotrigine, clonazepam, valproic acid, and even gabapentin. Currently, carbamazepine and oxcarbazepine are the first-line drugs of choice given a near 90% rate of efficacy with a more tolerable side effect-profile followed by phenytoin as a second-line agent.[1,7]

Percutaneous Ablative Techniques

Percutaneous chemoneurolysis

Chemoneurolysis for the treatment of TN with the use of alcohol injections into peripheral nerves was first introduced by Schloesser in 1904.[2] The side effects of this treatment, however, included temporary weakness of the muscles of mastication, transient anesthesia or paresthesias, and recurrence of TN after initial relief.[2,8] Over the years, in an attempt to provide more lasting effects, more toxic or caustic agents were entertained for injection into the Gasserian ganglion, uch as osmic acid, alcohol, and glycerol. ronically, the discovery of glycerol as a potential reatment was developed by chance while using lycerol to introduce tantalum dust into the trigemnal cistern.[9] This event led to the birth of percutaeous retrogasserian glycerol chemoneurolysis. However, all percutaneous procedures only ielded temporary relief with a higher likelihood of recurrence.[1,10]

ercutaneous radiofrequency lesioning

lectrocoagulation of the trigeminal nerve was irst described and attempted by Rethi in 1913.[8] n 1931, Kirschner[11] developed a stereotactic approach for insertion of an insulated needle hrough the foramen ovale for electrocoagulation of the Gasserian ganglion using monopolar cautery. Radiofrequency thermal lesioning of the preganglionic trigeminal rootlets was introduced n 1974 by Sweet and Wepsic.[12] They combined various measures to control the current delivery ncluding short-acting anesthetic drugs, electrical stimulation, and temperature monitoring and paved the way to improve the efficacy and safety of the procedure. Since their initial description of he technique, many prominent neurosurgeons such as Nugent,[13] Rovit,[14] and Tew and Taha[15] have worked to further improve the approach, such as modifications in the electrode type that allowed for more selective lesioning of the sensory ibers of the nerve and the repetition of small, less dense lesions during one treatment session. Of all he percutaneous techniques, radiofrequency esioning is associated with longer duration of pain relief. However, it also carries a higher risk of facial numbness, corneal anesthesia, keratitis, and anesthesia dolorosa.[16] There is also a higher risk of complications for repeat procedures.

Percutaneous balloon microcompression

n 1983, Mullan and Lictor[17] introduced percutaneous balloon compression of the Gasserian ganglion. The procedure involved threading a Fogarty balloon catheter into the foramen ovale and the trigeminal cistern. Inflation of the balloon caused mechanical injury to the trigeminal ganglion and the preganglionic rootlets. Initial complications included transient ipsilateral masseter and pterygoid muscle weakness. Mullan and Lictor's technique was further refined in 1996 by Brown and colleagues,[18] who developed the idea of using a blunt stylet following initial skin penetration to avoid vascular injury. However, despite the advances in the use of percutaneous balloon compression, several limitations exist, including bradycardia and brief hypotension caused by the trigeminocardiac reflex, postoperative numbness, and temporary weakness in the muscles of mastication, which can occur in up to 66% of patients.[16]

Stereotactic Radiosurgery

Initial efforts at irradiation of the Gasserian ganglion in the 1890s yielded disappointing results.[2] In 1971, Lars Leksell[19] used stereotactically focused radiation targeted to the trigeminal ganglion in order to treat a small number of patients with trigeminal neuralgia. However, with the advent of stereotaxis and better targeting over time at the dorsal root entry zone,[19,20] retrogasserian gamma knife surgery (GKS) has become a safe and efficacious modality for the treatment of TN for both first- and second-line treatment given its low side-effect profile, avoidance of open surgery, and patient satisfaction.[21,22] This involves using photon energy to create a destructive lesion using focused radiation to injure the sensory root. Although initial pain relief can be achieved in up to 90% of cases, patients typically do not experience immediate posttreatment pain relief because of a lag time ranging from 1 to 3 months.[23] One of the side effects is facial numbness, ranging from 20% to 32%.[16] One of the challenges of GKS is the long-term durability of pain relief. In a study by Dhople and colleagues,[24] freedom from pain goes down by 50% by 5 years. With a median follow-up of 5.6 years in 102 patients treated with GKS, 64% remained pain free and off medications, whereas 19% remained in severe pain with inadequate pain control. Nevertheless, GKS for TN may be the procedure of choice for nonsurgical candidates or patients with multiple medical comorbidities for whom open surgery carries increased risk.

Open Surgical Management of Trigeminal Neuralgia

Nerve sectioning

Treatments for TN have existed for as long as the condition itself was recognized.[1] Surgical treatment directly targeting the trigeminal ganglion was first reported by Carnochan in 1858.[2] Carnochan's theory was further refined over the next few decades by various surgeons from around the world, namely Rose in London[2]; Andrews in Chicago[2]; and Horsley, Taylor, and Coleman.[25] In 1892, Hartley (**Fig. 2**A) and Krause (**Fig. 2**B) independently described an extradural, subtemporal, middle fossa approach for Gasserian ganglionectomy. Through the Hartley-Krause approach, the nerves were divided at the foramen ovale and the foramen rotundum and excised to a point back beyond the Gasserian ganglion (**Fig. 3**). Spiller and Frazier further refined this technique by

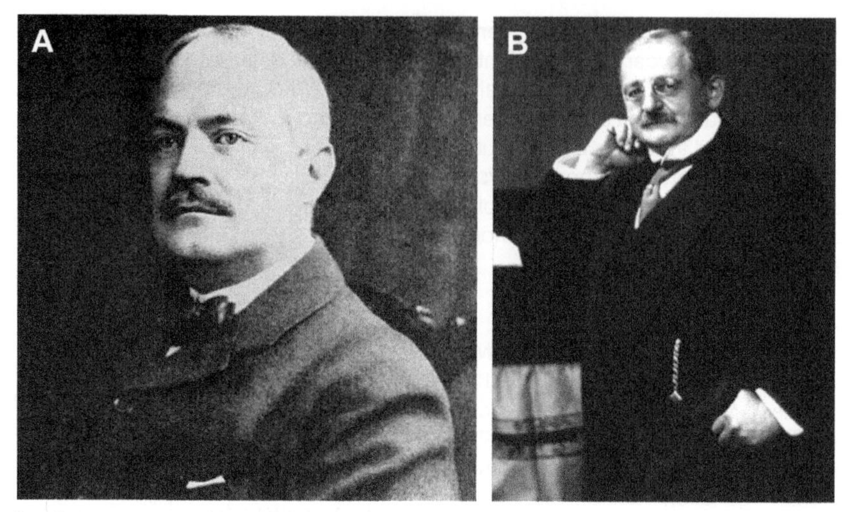

Fig. 2. Portraits of surgeons, Frank Hartley (*A*) and Fedor Krause (*B*), who described an extradural, subtemporal, middle fossa approach for Gasserian ganglionectomy in 1892. ([*A*] *Reprinted from* Stookey B, Ransohoff J. Trigeminal neuralgia: its history and treatment. Springfield (IL): Charles C. Thomas; 1959; and [*B*] *Courtesy of* National Library of Medicine, Bethesda, MD.)

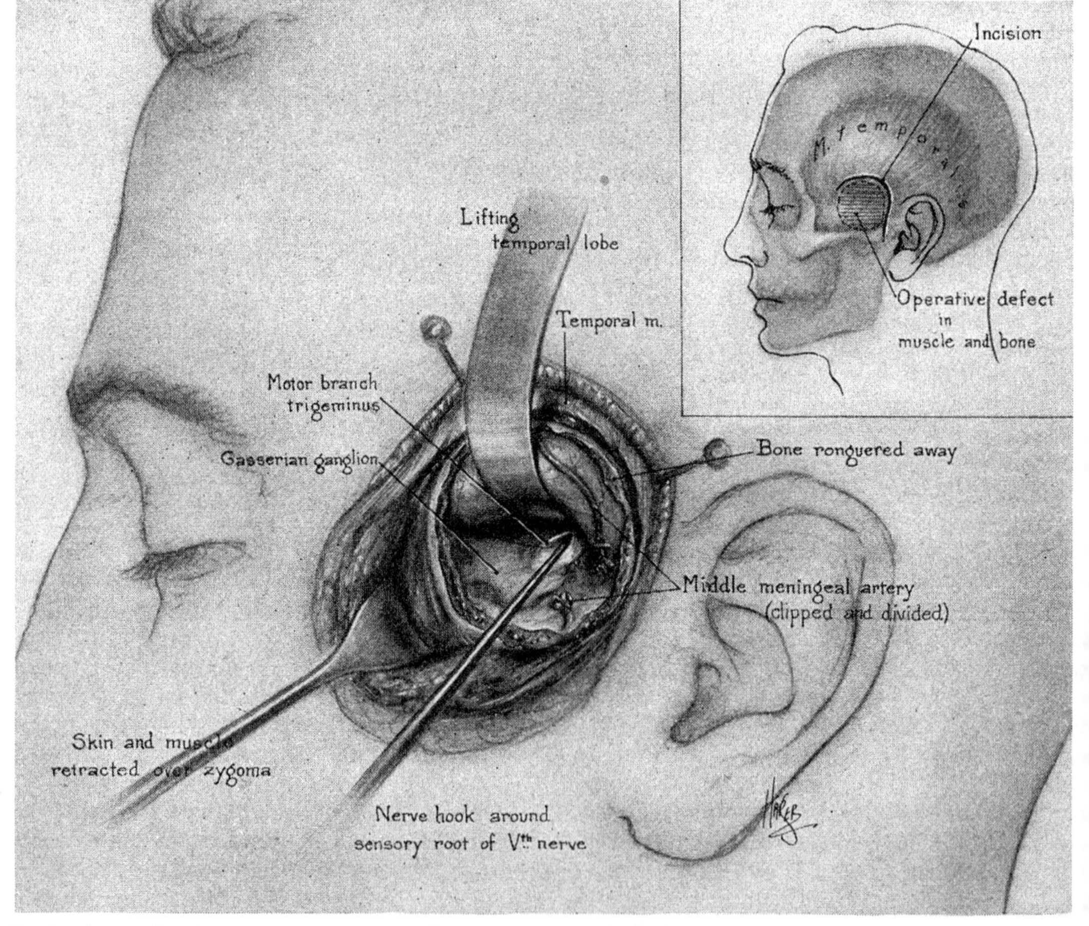

Fig. 3. The Hartley-Krause approach as modified by Frazier and Spiller. The temporal lobe has been retracted upward, and the nerve hook is around the sensory root, while the Gasserion ganglion can be visualized anteriorly; the motor root is found more medially. (*Reprinted from* Dandy WE. The brain. In: Walters W, Ellis FH Jr, editors. Lewis–Walters practice of surgery, vol. XII. Hagerstown (MD): W.F. Prior Co; 1963. p. 1–671.)

sparing the upper portion of the ganglion and the first branch of the trigeminal nerve to decrease the risk of corneal ulceration. In 1921, Frazier declared that "the problem of trigeminal neuralgia had been mastered."[26]

By 1928, Cushing, Frazier, and Stookey had all advanced the technique by selectively sectioning only the affected fibers in the dorsal trigeminal root. Thus the Spiller-Frazier procedure became the established and preferred surgical treatment for TN for close to 50 years. Although it was associated with an astonishingly high rate of facial paralysis and the feared complication of keratitis, many of the great neurosurgeons of the day hailed it as a safe and effective procedure. In this early era of neurosurgery, any procedure shown to be moderately effective with "acceptable" risks was quickly adopted. At the time, most neurosurgical operations still carried about a 50% risk of mortality.[2] Therefore, when Spiller and Frazier revealed their operation was associated with little morbidity and decent outcomes, it was rapidly accepted.

Walter Dandy (**Fig. 4**), however, was not particularly convinced of the effectiveness of the Spiller-Frazier approach. Having done hundreds of such cases, he found that facial paralysis, facial anesthesia, and other serious complications were occurring too often. During the 1920s, Dandy developed a suboccipital, cerebellar surgical approach (**Fig. 5**), which involved complete or partial sectioning of the sensory root of the trigeminal nerve within the posterior fossa instead of the middle fossa (**Fig. 6**). Dandy emphasized the importance of locating the junction of the transverse and sigmoid sinuses and obtaining an adequate dural exposure to approach the fifth cranial nerve.[26] Initially, Dandy performed a complete neurectomy of the sensory root. Later, through experimentation, he modified his technique to perform only a partial sectioning of the root (see **Fig. 6**). He found that this technique allowed for the retention of sensation to touch. Even more important to Dandy was that the operation was "relatively bloodless" and had a much lower risk of facial paralysis as the approach targeted the furthest part of the Gasserian ganglion from the facial nerve and trigeminal motor root.[27]

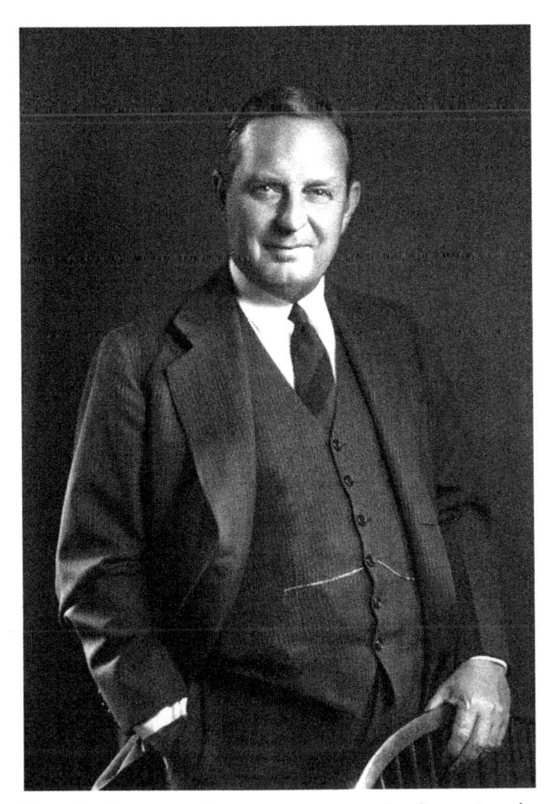

Fig. 4. Renowned neurosurgeon, Walter Dandy. (*Courtesy of* Mary Ellen Marmaduke.)

Evolution of microvascular decompression

Dandy's observation of neurovascular compression By the 20th century, partial sectioning of the nerve was found to be an effective approach to relieve the pain.[2,28–30] Currently, TN is a treatable condition, and the gold standard treatment for medically refractory TN is the microvascular decompression (MVD) procedure. Few operations in neurosurgery provide the satisfaction of complete cure and immediate results as the MVD procedure does for TN. MVD has a success rate approaching 90% with long-term durability.[7,31,32] Conceptually, MVD involves separating the trigeminal ganglion from the offending vascular structure that initially compressed or placed pressure on the trigeminal root. However, given its convoluted history, the discovery and acceptance of this concept was anything but simple.

Walter Dandy first published his surgical approach in 1925 as a preliminary report in the Johns Hopkins Hospital Bulletin.[33] He thought little of the approach at the time, writing later, "At that time, I entertained little enthusiasm for the procedure as a routine measure in treating persons with tic douloureux because the method [Spiller-Frazier method] then in use was so safe."[25] However, as Dandy started to use his procedure to a greater extent, he noticed a difference. He observed that he did not see the complications related to corneal and facial anesthesia and motor root injury with his approach. By 1927, Dandy had completely abandoned the Frazier method in favor of his own.

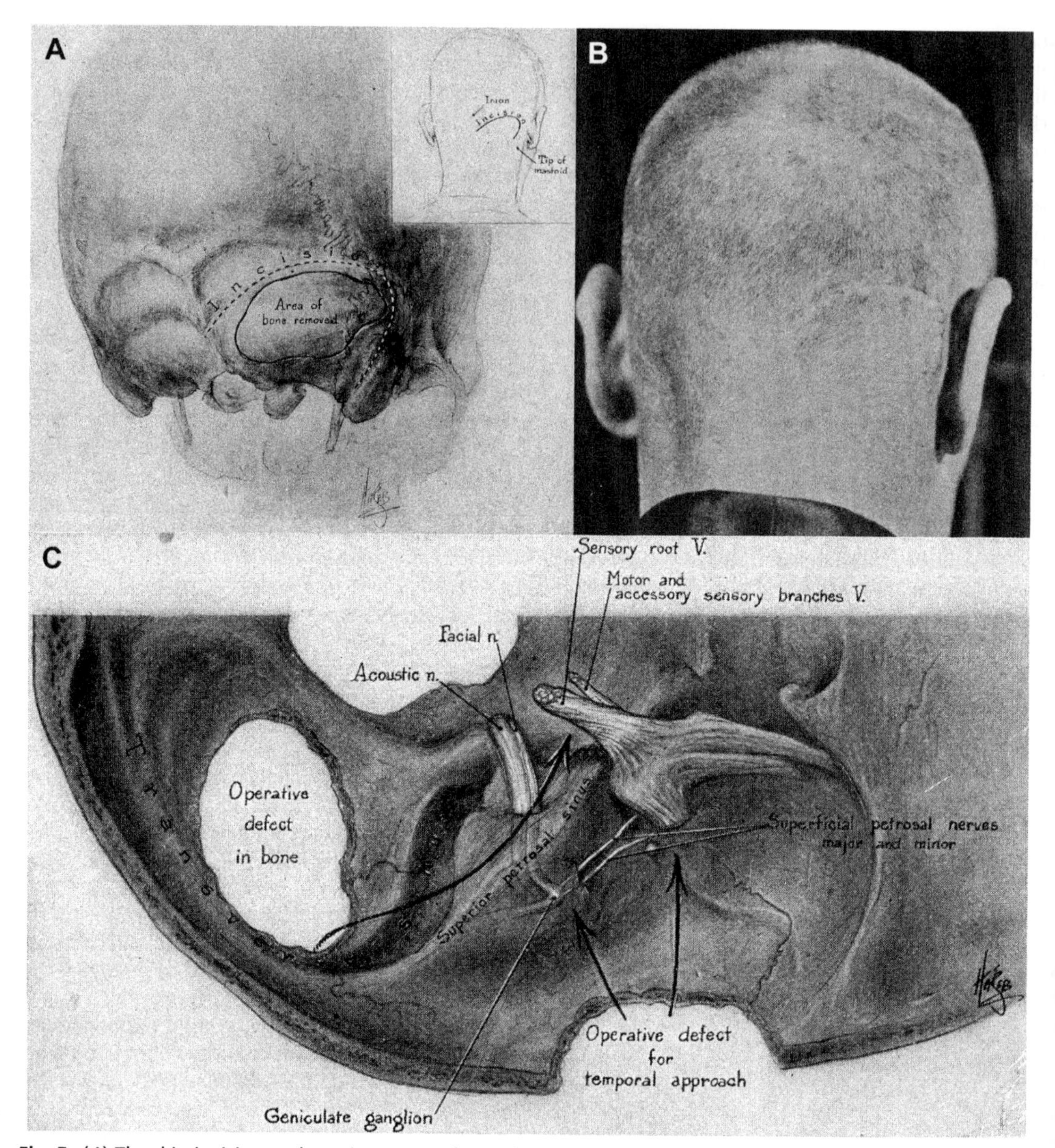

Fig. 5. (*A*) The skin incision and craniotomy performed with Dandy's suboccipital cerebellar approach to access the trigeminal root. (*B*) Healed skin incision with Dandy's surgical approach. (*C*) Operative approach and exposure created by both the temporal or middle fossa approach classically done by Hartley and Krause versus the suboccipital or posterior fossa approach advocated by Dandy. (*Reprinted from* Dandy WE. The brain. In: Walters W, Ellis FH Jr, editors. Lewis–Walters practice of surgery, vol. XII. Hagerstown (MD): W.F. Prior Co; 1963. p. 1–671.)

In 1929, Dandy published the description of his technique along with his results from his first 88 patients.[25] It this publication, Dandy casually commented that he occasionally observed random arterial loops to obstruct his view of the sensory root of the trigeminal ganglion. Unbeknownst to Dandy, he had performed a MVD of the trigeminal nerve root for the first time in neurosurgical history. At this point, however, Dandy did not quite understand the importance of the vascular loops that he occasionally encountered upon exposure of the Gasserian ganglion. In 1932, Dandy published his landmark report, which reviewed more than 250 consecutive cases of TN treated by trigeminal neurectomies using the cerebellar approach.[34] This time, he was even more

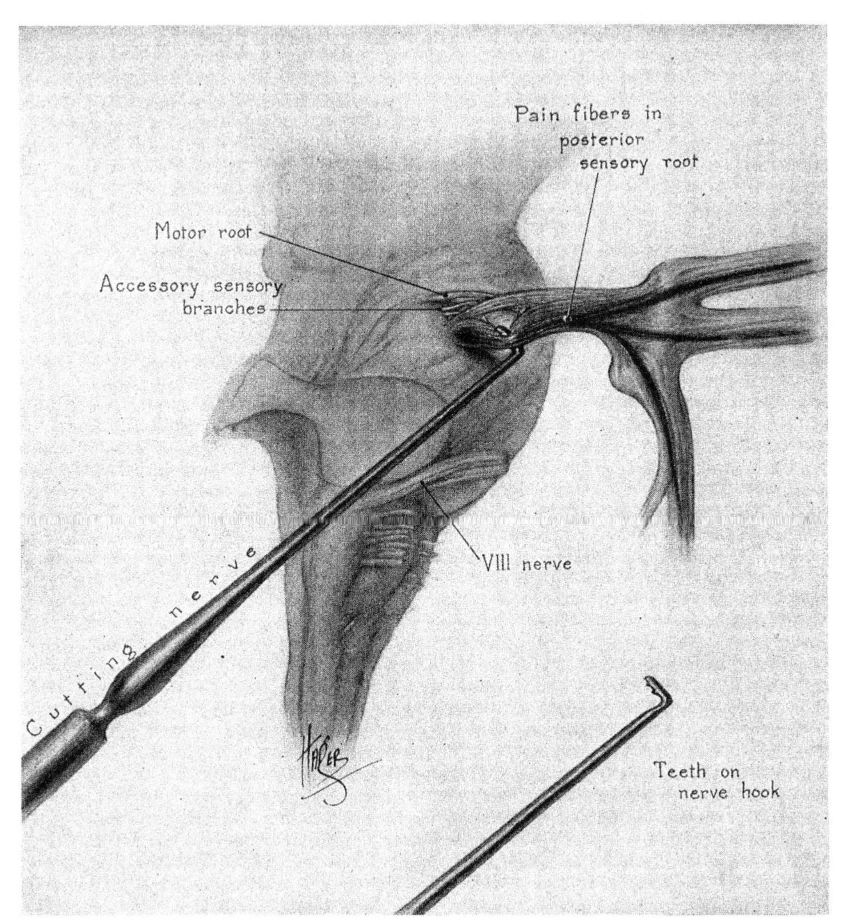

Fig. 6. Diagram shows the method of partial sectioning of the root. By only sectioning the 3 branches of the nerve located in the posterior half of the sensory root (as depicted by the dark fibers in the nerve hook), the pain of trigeminal neuralgia could be relieved while still maintaining the sensation of touch. (*Reprinted from* Dandy WE. The brain. In: Walters W, Ellis FH Jr, editors. Lewis–Walters practice of surgery, vol. XII. Hagerstown (MD): W.F. Prior Co; 1963. p. 1–671.)

convinced that something was amiss with the mass effect and pressure he often found exerted on the trigeminal nerve by various neighboring tumors or vascular pathology. Having seen it all too often, Dandy finally believed he had discovered a possible cause for TN. He wrote about the many occasions in which he visualized that the shape of the nerve was altered due to compression by an artery (**Fig. 7**). And he so boldly stated, "This I believe is the cause of tic douloureux."

However, Dandy's radical discoveries came at a time when the neurosurgical community had been convinced of the efficacy and safety of the Spiller-Frazier approach. As a result, it seemed unlikely that the field would accept another theory with open arms even if the procedure had been reported with modest results.[26] Marching forward undeterred, Dandy had completed 500 cases by 1934. In an analysis of 215 cases, of which he himself had personally written the operative note, entitled Concerning the Cause of Trigeminal Neuralgia,[35] Dandy found, that in 60% of cases, there was always some sort of mass effect on the root entry zone of the trigeminal nerve. In most cases, this was caused by the superior cerebellar artery (66 times) or petrosal vein (30 times) found to be present on the nerve. In fewer cases, he observed tumors and aneurysms as the source of neurovascular compression. Even in cases without gross findings, Dandy held on to the conviction that something there was still compressing the nerve.

Of course Dandy's hypotheses later proved to be remarkably accurate. Why he did not test these hypotheses at the time remains unknown. It is also significant to note that Dandy recorded these observations without the aid of a surgical

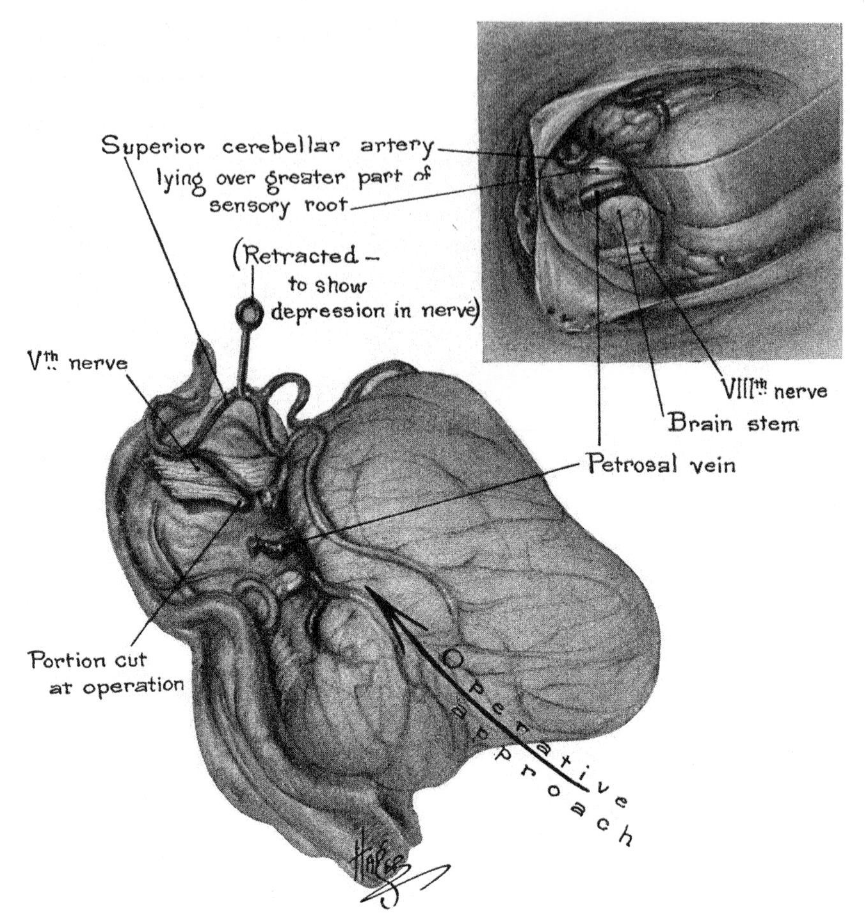

Fig. 7. Superior cerebellar artery as it contacts the trigeminal root and causing compression of the nerve root, one of the potential causes of trigeminal neuralgia. (*Reprinted from* Dandy WE. The brain. In: Walters W, Ellis FH Jr, editors. Lewis–Walters practice of surgery, vol. XII. Hagerstown (MD): W.F. Prior Co; 1963. p. 1–671.)

microscope, an incredible feat, as many of these vascular structures are indistinguishable to the naked eye. The small size of the venous and arterial structures account for the fact that Dandy reported only finding compression of the trigeminal nerve by arteries or veins in less than half of his cases. After 1934, although he continued to use his operative technique for his patients, Dandy never published another article on TN, and by the 1940s his approach had been largely forgotten for close to 18 years.[26]

Resurrection of a repressed theory In the early 1950s, Dandy's ideas would gain new life, not in the United States, but in Europe. Palle Taarnhøj, a young neurosurgeon from the University Hospital (Rigshospitalet) in Copenhagen, Denmark would be instrumental in reviving Dandy's hypothesis. The Taarnhøj procedure came to basically involve a modification of the Spiller-Frazier approach to the ganglion through the temporal route in which the middle fossa would be exposed intradurally through a small temporal craniectomy, and the dura would then be divided widely over the posterior part of the ganglion and root.[36,37] Taarnhøj's work was met with great enthusiasm in the neurosurgical world. The possibility of a cure for TN without the complications of facial paralysis or paresthesia was attractive to many surgeons at the time. In 1954, Taarnhøj published a series of 70 TN patients treated with his decompressive surgery and reported complete remission of pain in 41 of the patients. Recurrences were noted in only 9 cases. No patients suffered from permanent facial anesthesia or facial paralysis.[38,39]

Across the Atlantic, Taarnhøj's work in Denmark was being closely watched by W. James Gardner at the Cleveland Clinic (**Fig. 8**). When Taarnhøj published his preliminary results in 1952, Gardner quickly grasped the paradigm shift it caused. He

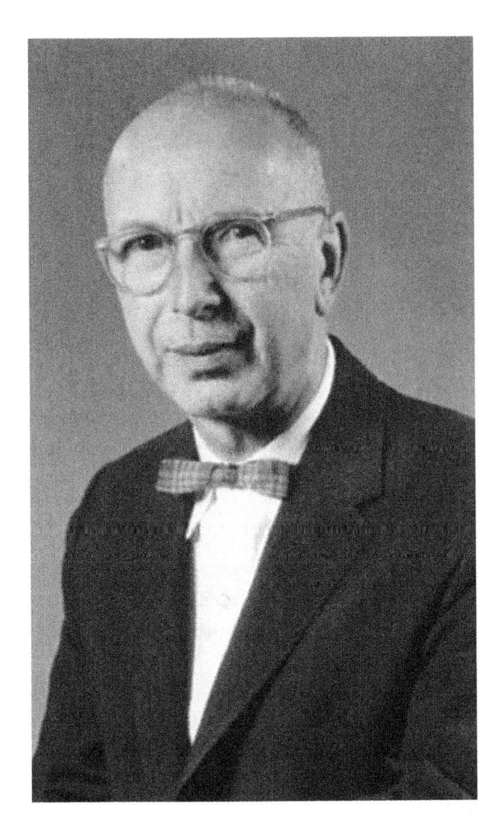

Fig. 8. Dr W James Gardner of the Cleveland clinic. (*Reprinted from* Dohn DF. W. James Gardner: a biographical sketch. Surg Neurol 1991;35:5–7.)

adopted the method and reported his first 9 patients by 1953.[40] Gardner practiced decompression using the combined extradural approach of Frazier and Dandy's posterior fossa approach. Once the dura was opened anterior to the petrous bone, the dural sheath protecting the sensory root was cut through the petrosal sinus. Once the sensory root was freed from the dural sheath, the nerve was "gently brushed with a cotton pledget, and irrigated with Ringer's solution."[40] Gardner continued to work at a furious pace over the next few years, working on hundreds of cases. In a landmark report published in 1959, Gardner and Miklos[41] detailed the outcomes of decompression of the sensory root performed on 112 patients treated between 1953 and 1955. Gardner's own case series of 100 patients with 3- to 5-year follow-up (also known as the Cleveland series) was compared with that of Taarnhøj's 100-patient series (known as the Copenhagen series). When the results of both series were combined, it was concluded that 62% of patients had immediate, complete, and lasting relief in their pain.

Gardner's extensive experience treating patients with TN led him to conclude that the underlying cause of TN was the "approximation of intact axis cylinders in the nerve root,"[4] and the approximation may be the result of the loss of myelin or of pressure and of aging. Anomalous arteries, aneurysms, basilar impressions, ipsilateral posterior fossa neoplasms, and other physiologic abnormalities might cause this damaging pressure on the trigeminal root. Gardner explained, "a prolonged period of gentle compression appears to be necessary to produce the pathophysiological state responsible for the paroxysms." Like Dandy, Gardner was instrumental in establishing the rationale behind and technique for decompression surgery of the trigeminal ganglion. However, just like Dandy, Gardner's exceptional surgical talents could not make up for the lack of an operating microscope to definitively prove the vascular compression hypothesis and further perfect the MVD procedure.

Acceptance of the Jannetta procedure The final development of the classic MVD procedure thus fell to Peter J. Jannetta (**Fig. 9**). Through this experience, Jannetta became convinced of the utility of the microscope in neurosurgical cases. By using

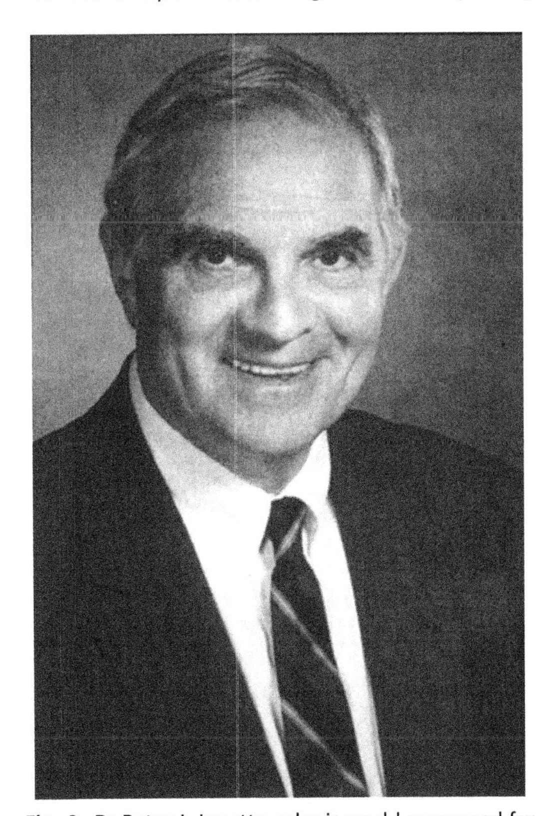

Fig. 9. Dr Peter J. Janetta, who is world renowned for his work in advancing the techniques of microvascular decompression for the treatment of trigeminal neuralgia. (*From* Cole CD, Liu JK, Apfelbaum RL. Historical perspectives on the diagnosis and treatment of trigeminal neuralgia. Neurosurg Focus 2005;18(5):E4.)

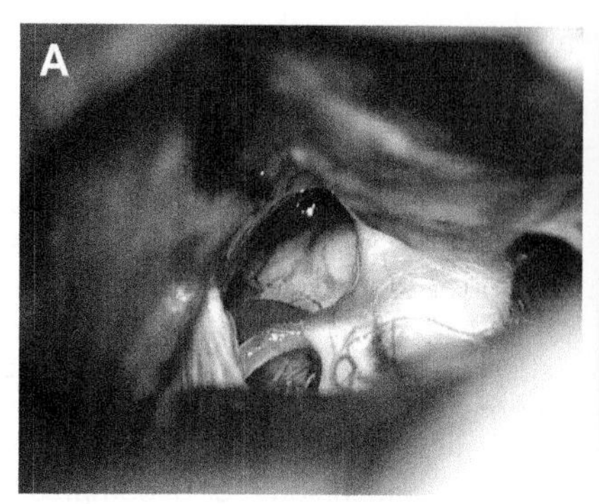

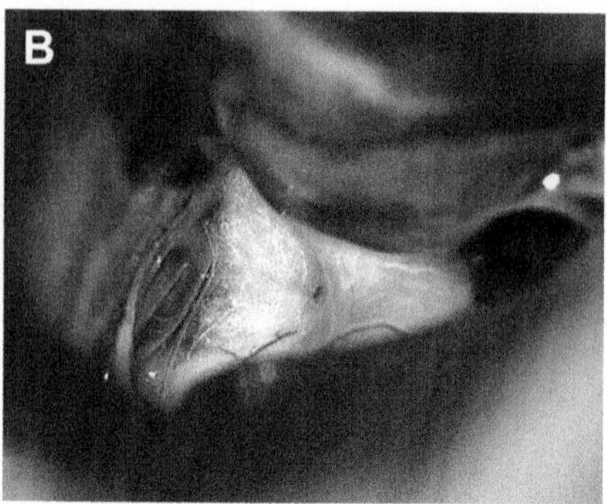

Fig. 10. Microscopic visualization with a right retrosigmoid approach for microvascular decompression for trigeminal neuralgia. (*A*) The superior cerebellar artery can been seen compressing the trigeminal nerve at the root entry zone. (*B*) With careful arachnoid dissection, this vessel loop is carefully mobilized away from the nerve, and the nerve is padded with a Teflon sponge to complete the decompression. (© James K. Liu, MD, with permission.)

the operating microscope Jannetta was able to prove that TN was often associated with arterial or venous vascular compression, strategically located at the root entry zone, where central myelin merges into peripheral myelin. This finding led to localized demyelination and altered physiology within the trigeminal system, which has been described as neural short-circuiting. Jannetta refined his technique over the ensuing decade, eventually favoring a posterior fossa approach to the trigeminal root. At the time of visualization of the offending blood vessel, he would make use of Teflon padding to separate the blood vessel from the trigeminal nerve (**Fig. 10**). He chose Teflon because it was easy to manipulate and promoted minimal arachnoid scarring. Jannetta even operated on many of Gardner's old patients. It turned out that Gardner's preference of Gelfoam (Pfizer, New York, NY) would result in recurrence of symptoms in several of his earlier patients, as the Gelfoam slowly reabsorbed over time.

Nevertheless, it seemed that even in the 1990s, the scientific community needed convincing, and Jannetta would provide it in satisfying fashion. With the advent of the surgical microscope, Jannetta was able to view arteries and veins that were almost impossible to observe by the naked eye, even to most acute and skilled neurosurgeons, such as Dandy. At the time when Jannetta first observed arterial and venous compression of the trigeminal nerve, he was unaware of Dandy's and Gardner's published findings and surgical techniques. He later used the work of Dandy and Gardner and his own personal observations to build a strong claim for the rationale of MVD surgery. While reviewing Gardner's case studies, Jannetta was able to hone his own ideas and put forth a greater arsenal of evidence for the effectiveness of MVD. In 1996, 3 decades after his original MVD operation, Jannetta published the results of his series of 1185 patients treated with MVD at the Presbyterian University Hospital in Pittsburgh between 1972 and 1991.[31] The initial success rate was 82% for complete relief with an additional 16% having partial relief for a combined initial success rate of 98%. At 10-year follow-up, 68% of patients reported excellent or good relief, whereas the remaining 32% experienced recurrent symptoms.[31]

It was with great patience and persistence that Peter Jannetta finally convinced the neurosurgical community to test his observations. Over time, long-term studies documented the durability of the MVD procedure, and it has now become the open procedure of choice for treatment for TN. Jannetta subsequently extended his observations to other cranial nerves and defined other neurovascular compression syndromes that were also treated by MVD, such as hemifacial spasm and glossopharyngeal neuralgia.[42,43] Jannetta's most valued contribution to the development of MVD surgery is perhaps best summarized by Shelton in his book, "Walter Dandy may have understood principally the same thing, but only Peter Jannetta managed to get the rest of the profession to believe it."[26]

SUMMARY

The predicament of trigeminal neuralgia that once perplexed many neurosurgeons has now become a curable condition, although its potential etiologies continue to intrigue clinicians. The vascular compression etiology of tic douloureux was initially noted by Dandy, later supported by the work of Taarnhøj and Gardner, and confirmed by Jannetta with the advent of the operative microscope. Since its earliest descriptions for the treatment of trigeminal neuralgia, the concept of microvascular decompression surgery has a ich history. It serves as a great example of how he field of neurosurgery continues to evolve remendously over generations with increasing knowledge of the root causes of various conditions and further advancements in surgical echnique.

REFERENCES

1. Cole CD, Liu JK, Apfelbaum RI. Historical perspectives on the diagnosis and treatment of trigeminal neuralgia. Neurosurg Focus 2005;18(5):E4.
2. Stookey B, Ransohoff J. Trigeminal neuralgia: its history and treatment. Springfield (IL): Charles C. Thomas; 1959.
3. Fothergill J. Of a painful affection of the face. Society of physicians in London: medical observations and inquiries. vol. 5; 1773. p. 129–42.
4. Hutchinson B. Cases of tic douloureux successfully treated. London: Longmans; 1820.
5. Napier L, Sen Gupta P. A peculiar neurological sequel to administration of 4:4'-diamidino-diphenylethylene (M & B 744). Ind Med Gaz 1942;77:71–4.
6. Bergouignan M. Cures heureuses de neurologies essentielles par le dephenyl hydantoinate de sounde. Rev Laryngol Otol Rhinol 1942;63:34–41.
7. Liu JK, Apfelbaum RI. Treatment of trigeminal neuralgia. Neurosurg Clin N Am 2004;15(3):319–34.
8. Wilkins R. Trigeminal neuralgia: historical overview, with emphasis on surgical treatment. In: Burchiel K, editor. Surgical management of pain. New York: Thieme; 2002. p. 288 301.
9. Hakanson S. Trigeminal neuralgia treated by the injection of glycerol into the trigeminal cistern. Neurosurgery 1981;9(6):638–46.
10. Lunsford LD, Apfelbaum RI. Choice of surgical therapeutic modalities for treatment of trigeminal neuralgia: microvascular decompression, percutaneous retrogasserian thermal, or glycerol rhizotomy. Clin Neurosurg 1985;32:319–33.
11. Kirschner M. Zur elektrochirurgie. Langenbecks Arch Klin Chir 1931;167:761–8.
12. Sweet W, Wepsic J. Controlled thermocoagulation of trigeminal ganglion and rootlets for differential destruction of pain fibers 1. Trigeminal neuralgia. J Neurosurg 1974;40:143–56.
13. Nugent G. Radiofrequency treatment of trigeminal neuralgia using a cordotomy-type electrode. A method. Neurosurg Clin N Am 1997;8:41–52.
14. Rovit RL. Percutaneous radiofrequency thermal coagulation of the gasserian ganglion. In: Rovit RL, Murali R, Jannetta PJ, editors. Trigeminal neuralgia. Baltimore (MD): Williams & Wilkins; 1990. p. 109–36.
15. Tew J, Taha J. Percutaneous rhizotomy in the treatment of intractable facial pain (trigeminal, glossopharyngeal, and vagal nerves). In: Schmidek H, Sweet W, editors. Operative neurosurgical techniques: indications, methods and results. 3rd edition. Philadelphia: WB Saunders; 1996. p. 1409–18.
16. Tatli M, Satici O, Kanpolat Y, et al. Various surgical modalities for trigeminal neuralgia: literature study of respective long-term outcomes. Acta Neurochir (Wien) 2008;150(3):243–55.
17. Mullan S, Lichtor T. Percutaneous microcompression of the trigeminal ganglion for trigeminal neurlagia. J Neurosurg 1983;59(6):1007–12.
18. Brown J, Chittum C, Sabol D, et al. Percutaneous balloon compression of the trigeminal nerve for treatment of trigeminal neuralgia. Neurosurg Focus 1996;1(2):e4.
19. Leksell L. Stereotaxic radiosurgery in trigeminal neuralgia. Acta Chir Scand 1971;137:311–4.
20. Rand RW. Leksell Gamma Knife treatment of tic douloureux. Neurosurg Clin N Am 1997;8:75–8.
21. Nanda A, Javalkar V, Zhang S, et al. Long term efficacy and patient satisfaction of microvascular decompression and gamma knife radiosurgery for trigeminal neuralgia. J Clin Neurosci 2015;22(5):818–22.
22. Regis J, Tuleasca C, Resseguier N, et al. Long-term safety and efficacy of Gamma Knife surgery in classical trigeminal neuralgia: a 497-patient historical cohort study. J Neurosurg 2016;124: 1079–87.
23. Urgosik D, Liscak R, Novotny J, et al. Treatment of essential trigeminal neuralgia with gamma knife surgery. J Neurosurg 2005; 102(Suppl):29–33.
24. Dhople A, Adams J, Maggio W, et al. Long-term outcomes of Gamma Knife radiosurgery for classic trigeminal neuralgia: implications of treatment and critical review of the literature. Clinical article. J Neurosurg 2009;111(2):351–8.
25. Dandy WE. An operation for the cure of tic douloureux: partial section of the sensory root at the pons. Arch Surg 1929;18(2):687–734.
26. Shelton ML. Working in a very small place: the making of a neurosurgeon. 1st Vintage Books edition. New York: Vintage Books; 1990.
27. Pinkus RL. Innovation in neurosurgery: walter dandy in his day. Neurosurgery 1984;14(5):623–31.
28. Hartley F. I. Intracranial neurectomy of the fifth nerve. Ann Surg 1893;17(5):511–526.1.
29. Rosegay H. The krause operations. J Neurosurg 1992;76(6):1032–6.
30. Krause F. Resection des trigeminus innerhalf der Schadelholhle. Arch Klin Chir 1892;44:821–32.
31. Barker FG 2nd, Jannetta PJ, Bissonette DJ, et al. The long-term outcome of microvascular decompression for trigeminal neuralgia. N Engl J Med 1996;334(17):1077–83.
32. Sindou M, Leston J, Decullier E, et al. Microvascular decompression for primary trigeminal neuralgia: long-term effectiveness and prognostic

factors in a series of 362 consecutive patients with clear-cut neurovascular conflicts who underwent pure decompression. J Neurosurg 2007;107(6):1144–53.
33. Dandy WE. Section of the sensory root of the trigeminal nerve at the pons. Preliminary report of the operative procedure. Bull Johns Hopkins Hosp 1925;36:105.
34. Dandy WE. The treatment of trigeminal neuralgia by the cerebellar route. Ann Surg 1932;96(4):787–95.
35. Dandy WE. Concerning the cause of trigeminal neuralgia. Am J Surg 1934;24:447–55.
36. Taarnhoj P. Decompression of the trigeminal root and the posterior part of the ganglion as treatment in trigeminal neuralgia; preliminary communication. J Neurosurg 1952;9(3):288–90.
37. Taarnhoj P. A new operation for trigeminus neuralgia; decompression of the trigeminal root and the posterior part of the ganglion; preliminary report. Nord Med 1952;47(11):360–4 [in Undetermined Language].
38. Taarnhoj P. Trigeminal neuralgia and decompression of the trigeminal root. Surg Clin North Am 1956;1145–57.
39. Taarnhoj P. Decompression of the trigeminal root. J Neurosurg 1954;11(3):299–305.
40. Gardner WJ, Pinto JP. The tarrnhoj operation; relief of trigeminal neuralgia without numbness. Cleve Clin Q 1953;20(2):364–7.
41. Gardner WJ, Miklos MV. Response of trigeminal neuralgia to decompression of sensory root; discussion of cause of trigeminal neuralgia. J Am Med Assoc 1959;170(15):1773–6.
42. Moller AR, Jannetta PJ. Microvascular decompression in hemifacial spasm: intraoperative electrophysiological observations. Neurosurgery 1985;16(5):612–8.
43. Jannetta PJ. Outcome after microvascular decompression for typical trigeminal neuralgia, hemifacial spasm, tinnitus, disabling positional vertigo, and glossopharyngeal neuralgia (honored guest lecture). Clin Neurosurg 1997;44:331–83.

Percutaneous Procedures for the Treatment of Trigeminal Neuralgia

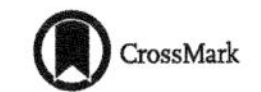

Matthew T. Bender, MD, Chetan Bettegowda, MD, PhD*

KEYWORDS

• Trigeminal neuralgia • Rhizotomy • Treatment

KEY POINTS

- Percutaneous procedures are safe and effective options for the management of trigeminal neuralgia.
- The best outcomes are seen after careful patient selection and counselling.
- An individualized treatment plan for each patient is essential for maximizing pain relief.

INTRODUCTION

Three types of percutaneous rhizotomy are currently used to treat trigeminal neuralgia (TN). Percutaneous balloon compression (PBC), glycerol rhizotomy (GR), and radiofrequency thermocoagulation (RFT) are all designed to interrupt afferent pain fibers by causing injury to the trigeminal nerve root or ganglion. Conceived in the early 20th century, several decades of experience with these relatively simple techniques have demonstrated their efficacy in offering immediate and durable pain relief, as well as overall safety.[1] Although microvascular decompression (MVD) has gained in popularity and the use of percutaneous rhizotomy has been on the decline,[2] these percutaneous techniques offer several important advantages. Partial sensory rhizotomy, an open procedure that can be performed if no vascular nerve compression is found during MVD, is not discussed in this paper.

HISTORY AND CONCEPTION

The first description of TN as a distinct disease entity dates back to 1688, by Fehr and Schmidt. More than a century later, the painful syndrome was localized to the trigeminal nerve, and eventually given the name that it bears today.[3] At the time, despite an intimate knowledge of the anatomy of the trigeminal nerve and ganglion, the pathophysiology of the disease was poorly understood. The first attempted treatment of TN occurred in 1910, when Harris injected the trigeminal ganglion with alcohol. Shortly afterward, in 1914, Hartel described a method for accessing the foramen ovale for percutaneous injections still in use today.[4,5] Only 2 years after Harris described his approach, Rethi attempted to treat TN by electrocoagulation of the trigeminal nerve and ganglion. Owing to limitations in electrode design, the procedure was associated with high complication rates as a result of unintended injury to the trigeminal nerve and surrounding structures.[3] Decades passed before Sweet and Wepsic, in 1974, described RFT of the trigeminal rootlets. With the use of short-acting anesthetic agents to allow for electrical stimulation and temperature monitoring, their method allowed for precise lesion creation.[6] Over the next few decades, Nugent further refined the technique with the use of a fine cordotomy-type electrode, and Tew and

Disclosure Statement: The authors have nothing to disclose.
Department of Neurosurgery, Johns Hopkins University School of Medicine, 600 North Wolfe Street, Phipps 118, Baltimore, MD 21287, USA
* Corresponding author.
E-mail address: cbetteg1@jhmi.edu

Neurosurg Clin N Am 27 (2016) 277–295
http://dx.doi.org/10.1016/j.nec.2016.02.005

Taha introduced curved thermistor-tipped electrodes, achieving high rates of pain relief with lower complication rates.[7,8]

The origins of GR date back to the late 19th century, when physicians injected various agents, including chloroform and osmic acid, next to nerve trunks with the goal of causing chemoneurolysis. Although reports indicate that this method was effective in producing pain relief, the effect was transient and often accompanied by significant weakness, sensory loss, and dysesthesias.[3] GR as it is exists today was developed somewhat serendipitously in 1981, when Hakanson and colleagues[9] were exploring the use of stereotactic radiotherapy as a treatment method for TN.[10,11] Glycerol, as a trivalent alcohol naturally present in human tissue, was used as the vehicle to suspend tantalum dust, and injected into the trigeminal cistern.[12] They found that injection of the carrier alone caused pain relief. Although it is thought that GR preferentially injures large myelinated fibers, the exact mechanism of action of glycerol is incompletely understood. Studies have suggested its hypertonicity, and more specifically, a rapid rate of change of intracellular osmolarity upon glycerol injection, results in axonal demyelination and fragmentation.[13–16] Although the procedure has been modified and updated in many ways, the core elements of the technique remains true to Hakanson's original method.

Balloon compression as a treatment for TN was discovered in the 1950s during investigations into scar tissue compressing the trigeminal nerve root or ganglion in the middle fossa as a cause of TN. In 1952, Taarnhøj described his method of decompression of the dorsal root of the trigeminal root, and Shelden and Pudenz reported a method for decompression of the second and third nerve divisions.[17,18] In working to decompress the trigeminal ganglion, they and others concluded that the effectiveness of their techniques in producing pain relief derived from the resultant injury to the posterior trigeminal root posterior to the ganglion. However, Shelden and colleagues[18] found that rubbing the posterior root was able to yield only transient pain relief. It was not until 1983, when Mullan and Lichtor[19] described compression of the trigeminal ganglion with a percutaneously inserted Fogarty balloon catheter, that trigeminal compression became a viable treatment option. Later studies in rabbits revealed that compression seems to preferentially affect the medium and large myelinated pain fibers, sparing small fibers, which allows for recovery of motor and sensory function, and theoretically, preservation of the corneal reflex.[20]

PATIENT SELECTION AND EVALUATION

The primary indication for percutaneous trigeminal rhizotomy remains Burchiel type 1 TN, or typical TN, an idiopathic condition in which patients experience episodic sharp or shooting electrical shock-like facial pain.[21] TN is a progressive disease, and without treatment, can transform to Burchiel type 2 TN, or atypical TN. Burchiel type 2 TN is characterized by more constant pain and is associated with sensory impairment. A trial of medical therapy with anticonvulsants is typically the initial treatment for TN, but there are no standardized guidelines regarding the minimum duration of medical therapy necessary before moving to an interventional strategy. Although some reports have suggested that trials of at least 2 anticonvulsants should be performed before surgical intervention, little evidence exists to support this notion.[22,23] Many patients experience initial pain relief with medication, but later develop breakthrough pain. Indeed, some studies have shown that more than 50% of patients with TN eventually undergo surgery.[24]

Several factors should be taken into consideration when making the choice of which surgical procedure to undertake. Percutaneous procedures are thought to be well-suited for elderly patients or those with multiple medical comorbidities for whom MVD would present a greater risk, or younger patients who wish to minimize their risk of postoperative facial numbness. However, age alone is not an absolute contraindication for craniotomy, because MVD has been shown to be well tolerated in patients older than 75 years.[1] RFT is not appropriate for patients who cannot tolerate an awake procedure or who are unable to cooperate with localization. There is a greater risk of the trigeminal depressor response and hypotension and bradycardia seen with PBC, making it less appropriate for some patients with cardiovascular disease. Each procedure allows for a varying degree division-specificity, but RFT can be used for more precise lesion creation than GR and PBC. Because of the supposed fiber-selective nature of PBC, many advocate the use of PBC for isolated first-division pain.[4] The comparative efficacy of percutaneous therapies, MVD, and stereotactic radiosurgery (SRS) is discussed elsewhere in this paper.

There are several patient subgroups who exhibit divergent outcomes from patients with typical TN. Atypical facial pain can refer to the both the quality or frequency of pain, or the underlying etiology, which can be iatrogenic, owing to postherpetic neuralgia, or in association with multiple sclerosis (MS). Although it is a nonspecific term, atypical pain has been associated with poorer outcomes in terms of symptom recurrence across several treatment modalities.[1,25,26] Management of patients with atypical facial pain will be discussed in detail (see Rahimpour S, Lad SP: Surgical Options for Atypical Facial Pain Syndromes, in this issue). Patients with MS also represent a unique subgroup, because they have a higher prevalence of TN compared with the general population.[27,28] The pathophysiologic link between the 2 conditions is incompletely understood, but TN is thought to result from combination of inflammatory and mechanical demyelination.[28–32]

SURGICAL TECHNIQUE

Percutaneous Balloon Rhizotomy

PBC is generally performed under general anesthesia. Entry into the foramen ovale can evoke the trigeminal depressor response, and the resultant hypotension and bradycardia can be significant. In preparation, a transcutaneous or transesophageal pacemaker is placed. Atropine is not given preoperatively to allow for monitoring of trigeminal compression intraoperatively, but should be prepared in the case of persistent bradycardia. The patient is positioned supine with a neck roll for 15° of extension. Hartel's anatomic landmarks are plotted, with 1 point inferior to the medial aspect of the ipsilateral pupil and a second point 3 cm anterior to the external auditory meatus, serving as the target trajectory. A third point 2.5 cm lateral to the ipsilateral oral commissure is the skin insertion point. A 14-gauge needle cannula is inserted and advanced along the target trajectory to the foramen ovale. A free hand technique is then used to direct the needle with a gloved finger inside the oral cavity to prevent violation of the buccal mucosa and to ensure the needle remains medial to the mandible. The needle is directed in a trajectory that bisects a triangle between the insertion point, the midpupillary line, and the marking 3 cm anterior to the external auditory meatus. Intraoperative visualization of needle and balloon placement is performed with lateral view fluoroscopy. Once the cannula is at the skull base, a submental view is obtained, and used to guide the cannula to the foramen ovale. Entry into the trigeminal cistern results in egress of cerebrospinal fluid, although this is not always observed.[7]

Engagement of the foramen ovale results in elicitation of the trigeminal depressor response, causing contraction of the masseter and pterygoid muscles. Under direct visualization of the foramen ovale, a straight guiding stylet is passed into the cannula. With an anteroposterior view, the stylet is directed toward the proximal entrance of the trigeminal fossa, the porus trigeminus, which is approximately 17 mm beyond the foramen ovale. Directing the stylet in the center of the porus is thought to treat second division or multidivision pain, whereas a lateral position treats third division pain, and medial, first division pain. Once the stylet has been advanced to the proper position, it is then removed, and a 4-F balloon catheter is introduced and advanced along the chosen trajectory to the target position. The balloon is inflated with 0.7 to 0.75 mL of iohexol to a target pressure of 1000 to 1200 mm Hg for 60 to 90 seconds. The balloon should take on a classic pear-shaped appearance, which reflects its position within the porus. During compression, the trigeminal depressor response is usually observed again and is a reflection of appropriate compression. The cannula and catheter can then be removed, and light manual pressure should be applied to the skin puncture site. An ice pack and sterile bandage is then applied to the site. The patient can be discharged home on the same day if stable, or observed overnight.

Radiofrequency Thermocoagulation

Because RFT requires patient cooperation during parts of the procedure, patients must be trained preoperatively to localize facial stimuli. Before the procedure, 0.4 mg of atropine is given intramuscularly to prevent bradycardia. As with PBC, the trigeminal depressor response can be evoked intraoperatively, but atropine can be preadministered because the response is not used for intraoperative monitoring. Induction is performed with a short-acting agent such as propofol, and patients are positioned as described for PBC. C-arm fluoroscopy is typically used to guide needle placement. A cannula with an obturator is then guided to the foramen ovale as noted previously, and its position confirmed with lateral view fluoroscopy. The obturator is then removed, and the electrode introduced. Caution should be taken to avoid placement of the electrode beyond 10 mm of the profile of the clivus, where the trochlear and abducens nerve lie. The patient can be awakened, and sensory and motor responses are tested. Locations to lesion are determined by detailed mapping to effect pain control and minimize sensory and motor side effects. Alternatively, the patient can be kept asleep throughout the surgery and the combination of fluoroscopy and nerve stimulation can be used to verify appropriate localization. The electrode is then removed, the thermocouple introduced to the previously chosen locations, and lesions are made at a maximum of 0.5 V at 5 and 75 cycles per second at 55 to 80°C for 30 seconds to 2 minutes. The electrode and cannula can then be withdrawn, pressure applied to the puncture site, and the site dressed. As with PBC, the patient can be discharged home on the same day if stable, or observed overnight.

Glycerol Rhizotomy

Induction is also performed with a short-acting agent such as propofol. The trigeminal depressor response can again be seen upon engagement of the foramen ovale and also upon injection of glycerol; atropine can be preadministered, as with RFT. C-arm fluoroscopy is used for guidance. A 20-gauge needle is used with Hartel's landmarks to guide the needle to the foramen ovale. Contrast-enhanced cisternography can be used to assess the trigeminal cistern and determine the necessary amount of glycerol to be injected. However, injection of 1 cm^3 air can also be used to outline the cistern. The head of the bed is then elevated to 60°, and glycerol is injected. The volume of glycerol typically varies from 0.25 to 0.40 mL; different volumes can be used to target specific divisions. For multidivision pain, injection of the full volume will treat all divisions. After the injection, the needle is removed, and the patient is awakened to remain in a sitting position for 2 hours so that the glycerol does not spill out of Meckel's cave. The patient can be discharged home on the same day if stable, or observed overnight.

Intraoperative Complications

Although the use of Hartel's landmarks to access the foramen ovale has been in widespread use for decades, the proximity of the foramen ovale to critical neurovascular structures should not be forgotten. The internal carotid artery can be punctured at the C2, C3, or C4 segments, typically resulting in pulsatile blood flow through the cannula. Serious injuries can result from inadvertent cannulation of the inferior orbital fissure or jugular foramen. Inappropriate placement of the cannula lateral to the trigeminal fossa in the subdural space medial to the temporal lobe can also result in intracranial hemorrhage. Skirving and Dan[4] noted 2 cases in which patients undergoing PBC experienced asystole upon engagement of the foramen ovale; in 1 case, the asystole resolved upon withdrawal of the needle, and the other patient required atropine. No mortality from the trigeminal depressor response during a percutaneous rhizotomy has been reported in the literature. Although all 3 of the percutaneous therapies are considered safe and associated with low mortality rates, there have been reports of intraoperative deaths during the procedures. For PBC, 2 deaths have been reported in the literature, in 1 case, from a punctured arteriovenous fistula, and in the second, from a brainstem hematoma.[33,34] No intraoperative deaths during GR or RFT have been reported.

PATIENT OUTCOMES

Percutaneous Balloon Compression

Rates of initial pain relief, which in most studies refers to complete pain relief without medications, are high in patients treated with PBC, ranging from 85% to 100% (**Table 1**).[4,35–44] One study of patients who required repeat procedures found a lower, but comparable, rate of pain relief at 83%.[40] Rates of pain recurrence range from 20% to 48%, again with 1 report of recurrence rates at 64% in a cohort with almost 90% patients who had previously undergone surgery.[41] Reporting of the time to recurrence also varies greatly across studies, with rates of recurrence at 5 years ranging from 19.2% to 29.5%. Postoperative facial numbness is present in the majority of patients, and typically resolves within 3 months.[4] The most commonly reported complications are masseter weakness or masticatory muscle weakness, and dysesthesias (**Table 2**).[22,45] Some degree of motor weakness is expected postoperatively owing to the impact of the procedure on large myelinated nerve fibers, with the rates of masseter weakness reported ranging from 10% to greater than 50%.[36,46,47] However, in the majority of cases, the weakness resolves within a few weeks to months.[35] Rates of dysesthesia range from 1.5% to 11.4%, and decrease with decreasing compression times. As with masseter weakness, in the majority of cases dysesthesia is minor and transient.[1] Early reports of PBC often highlight the low rates of corneal anesthesia associated with the procedure; indeed, in most contemporary reports of PBC, no patients experienced this complication.

Other complications that have been observed include hearing and olfactory disturbances, cranial nerve III, IV, and VI palsies, arteriovenous fistula development, meningitis, and herpes simplex labialis.[43,48] Catheter or balloon misplacement can result in injury to other cranial nerves, most commonly, the abducens, resulting in transient diplopia. Meningitis is a rare complication; the highest rate reported was 5%, and in the majority of series, no patients experienced meningitis. Herpes reactivation is common after procedures involving manipulation of the trigeminal nerve, and is typically mild and prophylactic antiviral therapy is typically not administered.[47] The development of more serious complications is extremely

Table 1
Selected studies of patient outcomes after percutaneous balloon compression

Study	n	No. of Procedures [a]	Follow-up Duration, (y)[b]	% Prior Procedure [c]	% MS	% Initial Relief [d]	% Recurrence [e]	Time to Recurrence [f]
Fraioli et al,[36] 1989	159	162	3	8.2	1.9	89.9	9.8	NR
Lichtor & Mullan,[35] 1990	100	104	(1–10)	37	3	100	28	20% at 5 y
Lobato et al,[37] 1990	144	155	(0.5–4.5)	43	2.1	100	9.7	NR
Brown et al,[38] 1993	50	50	3 (0.8–7.5)	52	10	94	26	1.5 y
Correa & Teixeira,[39] 1998	158	200	4	45.7	1.9	90	20	8.2% at 3 y
Skirving & Dan,[4] 2001	496	531	10.7	4	2.2	>99	31.9	19.2% in 5 y
Omeis et al,[40] 2008	29	41	4.1 (0.1–8.4)	100	7	83	45.5	0.6 y
Kouzounias et al,[41] 2010	47	47	1.7	89.4	36.2	85	64	1.4 y
Chen et al,[42] 2011	130	130	8.9	43.8	0	93.8	37.7	29.5% at 5 y
Bergenheim et al,[43] 2013	100	100	NR	48	23	90	48	2.3 y
Abdennebi & Guenane,[44] 2014	901	901	16.5 (0.5–27)	0.4	NR	92.7	27.8	NR

Abbreviations: MS, multiples sclerosis; NR, not recorded.

[a] Many studies report performing >1 procedure per patient; that is, after initial treatment failure, the authors performed another surgery on the same patient and reported long-term outcomes based on results after the second, or third, operation.

[b] Given as mean value ± standard deviation or (range), unless otherwise indicated.

[c] Other surgical interventions for trigeminal neuralgia, including other percutaneous procedures, microvascular decompression, or stereotactic radiosurgery.

[d] Defined as complete relief without medications, unless otherwise indicated.

[e] Defined as the percentage of patients who experienced pain recurrence during the follow-up period.

[f] Given as median time to recurrence or percentage of patients who experienced recurrence by a certain time postoperatively, unless otherwise indicated.

Data from Refs.[4,35–44]

Table 2
Selected studies of postoperative complications after percutaneous balloon compression

Study	n	% Dysesthesia	% Anesthesia Dolorosa	% Corneal Sensory Impairment[a]	% Diplopia	% Masticatory Weakness	% Meningitis
Fraioli et al,[36] 1989	159	6.9	0.6	0	0	6.9	NR
Lichtor & Mullan,[35] 1990	100	4	0	0	1	NR	0
Lobato et al,[37] 1990	144	19	0	NR	NR	12	NR
Brown et al,[38] 1993	50	NR	0	0	2	NR	3
Brown & Gouda,[99] 1997	141	3.5	0	0	NR	NA	NR
Correa & Teixeira,[39] 1998	158	NR	0	0	3	33	0.6
Skirving & Dan,[4] 2001	496	3.8	0	0	NR	NR	0
Chen et al,[42] 2011	130	1.5	0	2.3	1.5	6.2	0
Abdennebi & Guenane,[44] 2014	901	2.8	0	0.9	1.2	10.8	2.2

Abbreviations: MS, multiples sclerosis; NR, not recorded.
[a] Includes cases of corneal anesthesia.
Data from Refs.[4,35–39,42,44,99]

are after PBC. There is only 1 case of anesthesia dolorosa reported in the literature, and 3 cases of corneal keratitis.[40,41,49] One case of reversible blindness after PBC has been reported, owing to occlusion of orbital venous drainage to the cavernous sinus by the cannula, leading to increased intraocular pressure. With aggressive treatment with acetazolamide, visual acuity gradually returned.[48]

In terms of prognostic factors, achieving a pear-shaped balloon during compression has been highlighted by several studies as a key predictor of durable pain relief.[41,50] However, it remains a subjective criterion, and is ultimately a visual proxy for the position of the balloon catheter and the degree of compression. Objective variables that can be altered to change the degree of compression include the level of pressure and the duration of compression. Greater pressures, although associated with higher rates of pain relief, are also associated with added morbidity in the form of sensory alterations and motor weakness. Brown and Pilitsis[34] attempted to define the ideal level of compression with continuous balloon pressure monitoring, ultimately concluding that the optimal pressure ranged from 750 to 1250 mm Hg for 1.15 minutes. In addition, numerous studies have demonstrated that longer compression times do not seem to appreciably improve outcomes, while increasing rates of complications.[4,41,49,51,52] In the last few years, practice trends have shifted toward shorter compression times, with compression times of less than 60 seconds seeming to be adequate in achieving pain relief.

Radiofrequency Thermocoagulation

The goal of lesion production in RFT is to produce mild to moderate hypalgesia in the affected divisions, allowing for adequate pain control without causing significant sensory deficits. Although there is variability in the reported rates of initial pain relief, rates are generally relatively high, with most studies reporting greater than 95% complete pain resolution (**Table 3**).[7,36,53–57] Rates of pain control and the duration of pain relief consistently

Table 3
Selected studies of patient outcomes after radiofrequency thermocoagulation

Study	n	No. of Procedures	Follow-up Duration (y)	% Prior Procedure	% MS	% Initial Relief	% Recurrence	Time to Recurrence
Fraioli et al,[36] 1989	533	582	6.5	4.7	3.4	97.4	10	NR
Frank & Fabrizi,[53] 1989	700	700	3	NR	NR	NR	25	25% in 3 y
Broggi et al,[54] 1990	1000	1000	9.3 (5 14)	NR	NR	94.8	18.1	12.8% in 3 y
Scrivani et al,[55] 1999	215	215	2.7 (0.8–5.7)	NR	NR	92	27	NR
Tronnier et al,[56] 2001	206	206	14.0	NR	NR	NR	20	50% in 2 y, 75% in 4.5 y[a]
Kanpolat et al,[57] 2001	1600	2138	5.7 ± 5.5 (1–25)	27.5	NR	97.6	25.1	7.7% in <0.5 y, 17.4% in >0.5 y
Tew et al,[7] 2012	1200	1200	9 (1–21)	NR	NR	99.4	20	15% at 5 y, 7% from 5-10 y, 3% from 10-15 y[b]

Abbreviations: MS, multiples sclerosis; NR, not recorded.
[a] Long-term follow-up via questionnaires in which 206 out of 316 patients participated.
[b] Subset of 154 patients followed prospectively.
Data from Refs.[36,53–58]

correlate with the degree of sensory loss. Taha and colleagues,[58] in a prospective study of 154 patients, found that patients with anesthesia had the lowest rates of pain recurrence but the highest rates of dysesthesia. In contrast, patients with mild hypalgesia had the highest pain recurrence rates and the lowest rates of dysesthesia.

With high rates of durable pain relief, RFT is also associated with relatively higher rates of more severe side effects (**Table 4**). As for PBC, mild to moderate postoperative facial numbness and dysesthesia are common. Most cases of masseter weakness and diplopia seem to resolve by 6 to 12 months.[7] Rates of anesthesia dolorosa range from 0% to 12% in a series of 1600 patients, considerably higher than that for PBC.[57] In addition, although PBC is associated with extremely low rates of corneal anesthesia, this complication occurs at higher rates after RFT, from 1% to 20.3%.[7] Similarly, rates of masseter weakness are higher, ranging from 3% to 29% in 1 series. Other complications that are observed occasionally include keratitis, diplopia, meningitis, and carotid–cavernous fistula formation.[7] There has been 1 reported case of intracranial hemorrhage after RFT.[59] Few studies have examined predictors of outcomes after RFT. Kosugi and colleagues[60] found that outcomes were significantly better for patients with isolated third division pain, compared with second division and mutlidivision pain. Taha and colleagues[7] documented that their use of a curved rather than straight electrode allowed them to create more selective lesions to decrease rates of sensory complications.

Glycerol Rhizotomy

As noted, studies of GR vary greatly in their surgical technique and outcomes reporting. Reported rates of initial complete pain relief vary significantly, from 53.1% to 98%, as do rates of pain recurrence, from 13% 70% (**Table 5**).[25,36,43,61–69] Postoperative facial numbness is again common, and typically resolves within hours to days after the operation. Varying degrees of postoperative hypalgesia are also observed, with mild to moderate hypalgesia seen in up to 70% cases and typically lasting no more than 3 to 6 months.[14] As with other percutaneous treatments, facial numbness is positively correlated with pain relief. Severe hypalgesia and analgesia are rare, and patients who have undergone previous operations seem to be at greater risk.[70] The risk of anesthesia dolorosa and masticatory weakness are typically low,

Table 4
Selected studies of postoperative complications after radiofrequency thermocoagulation

Study	n	% Dysesthesia	% Anesthesia Dolorosa	% Corneal Sensory Impairment	% Diplopia	% Masticatory Weakness	% Meningitis
Fraioli et al,[36] 1989	533	15.2	1.5	20.3	0.2	3	NR
Frank & Fabrizi,[53] 1989	700	NR	0.6	1	0.1	8	NR
Broggi et al,[54] 1990	1000	5.2	1.5	20.3	0.5	10.5	NR
Scrivani et al,[55] 1999	215	8	1.8	2	0	29	0.9
Tronnier et al,[56] 2001	206	0.9	0	NR	NR	NR	NR
Kanpolat et al,[57] 2001	1600	1.0	12	5.7	0.88	4.1	0.06
Tew et al,[7] 2012	1200	20	1	6	1.2	16	0.2

Abbreviation: NR, not recorded.
Data from Refs.[36,53–58]

Table 5
Selected studies of patient outcomes after glycerol rhizotomy

Study	n	No. of Procedures	Follow-up Duration (y)	% Prior Procedure	% MS	% Initial Relief	% Recurrence	Time to Recurrence
Saini,[61] 1987	552	552	1–6	NR	NR	NR	NR	27.7% in 1 y, 40.9% in 2 y
Young,[62] 1988	162	173	0.5–5.6	9.3	NR	90.1	18.5	6%–7% in 1 y, 14.3% in 5 y
Fraioli et al,[36] 1989	32	32	5 y	15.6	6.3	53.1	13	NR
Fujimaki et al,[68] 1990	122	122	3.2–4.5	45	NR	78.7	50	2.7 y
North et al,[25] 1990	85	109	0.5–4.5	38.8	4.7	NR	NR	2.0 y
Steiger,[63] 1991	122	122	1.9 (1–8)	20	NR	84	23.0	59% in 5 y
Slettebo et al,[64] 1993	60	60	4.5 (1–9)	65	10	93	50	3.9 y
Bergenheim et al,[101] 1995	99	99	1.0	53	13.1	97	24.2	NR
Erdem & Alkan,[65] 2001	157	157	4.0	NR	NR	98	38.2	NR
Jagia et al,[69] 2004	100	140	0.5–3	NR	NR	66.1	NR	NR
Pollock,[66] 2005[a]	98	98	2.4 (0.3–4.3)	51	0	NR	28.3	1.4 y (mean)
Kouzounias et al,[75] 2010	101	120	NR	55	13	87	NR	1.3 y
Bender et al,[67] 2013	450	544	2.8 ± 3.3	21.6	0	69	70	2.1 y

Abbreviation: NR, not recorded.
[a] Included 7 patients with constant facial pain; outcomes from 92 patients with follow-up data.
Data from Refs.[25,36,41,43,61–69]

ranging from 0% to 5.0% and 0% to 4.1%, respectively (**Table 6**). Rates of corneal anesthesia are also considerably higher than those reported for PBC, ranging from 0% to 16%. Herpes reactivation seems to occur at higher rates, and was observed in 77% cases postoperatively in one series.[71]

North and colleagues[25] found that female sex, typical symptoms, successful prior medical therapy with carbamazepine, shorter duration of symptoms, and intraoperative cerebrospinal fluid return as all significantly associated with longer pain-free intervals. Although several early reports suggested that intraoperative cerebrospinal fluid egress was prognostic of improved outcomes, this association has not held up in more recent studies.[67,72] Other potential prognostic factors include lack of preoperative sensory deficits and lack of prior procedures, which seem to be predictive of initial pain relief; postoperative sensory deficits and intact preoperative facial sensation have been found to be predictive of durable pain relief. Pollock[66] found that nonconstant facial pain preoperatively, immediate pain upon glycerol injection, and new trigeminal deficits postoperatively were associated with improved outcomes. No association between use of cisternography and outcomes has been found.[14]

Study Limitations

The majority of studies of percutaneous rhizotomy are retrospective, and exhibit considerable variability in their patient populations, treatment technique, and outcomes reporting. Regarding the heterogeneous patient populations, studies include varying numbers of patients with atypical pain, MS, and bilateral TN, groups for which the outcomes are thought to be different from those with typical TN pain. Most series also include varying percentages of patients who are not treatment naïve in their cohorts. Although the general technique for each procedure is similar, each type of percutaneous rhizotomy has operator-dependent technical variations that limit comparisons. For example, with GR, the method for cisternography varies as does the volume of glycerin injected; for PBC, the level of pressure and duration compression, and for RFT, the type of electrode, delivery of energy, and location of lesioning.

A lack of standardization in pain relief outcomes and definition of complications also limits comparisons across the literature. Pain relief can be defined in a variety of ways: as a dichotomous variable, as either present or absent, or as improvement or lack of improvement after the operation, or based on subjective criteria such as patient satisfaction. An additional complicating factor is whether patients require medications postoperatively to achieve complete pain control. Efforts at standardization have been made, including the Barrow Neurologic Institute Pain Scale, which grades outcomes on a scale from I to V.[73] Furthermore, adverse events are often imprecisely defined, as hypalgesia or dysesthesia alone, without indicating the severity, division, or duration. Finally, a limitation intrinsic to any analysis of symptom recurrence is that reporting of recurrence depends heavily on the duration of follow-up. Although Kaplan-Meier analyses are able to in part control of such variability, the variability in outcomes reporting for TN makes defining the exact time of pain recurrence difficult. All of these factors hamper the use of single-modality studies in comparisons of outcomes across treatment modalities.

Comparative Treatment Efficacy

No randomized, controlled study comparing the 3 percutaneous therapies has been performed to date, and the few studies that do exist comparing outcomes across modalities are most often single-institution and retrospective (**Table 7**).[50,52,74–78] Fraioli and colleagues,[36] in comparing outcomes for PBC, RFT, and GR, recommended PBC as the first-line choice for percutaneous rhizotomy given its high efficacy rate and low complication rates. Kouzounias and colleagues[75] examined outcomes after PBC and GR, finding comparable rates of initial pain relief for each procedure as well as comparable times to recurrence. GR was associated with an overall complication rate of 11%, compared with 23% for PBC, with PBC cases more frequently complicated by masseter weakness, diplopia, and hearing and olfactory disturbances. They concluded that GR should be the first-line treatment; however, more patients undergoing PBC had previously experienced surgical intervention compared with those who underwent GR, which may explain the higher complication rate seen with PBC.[75] Asplund and colleagues[50] also compared PBC with GR, ultimately recommending PBC as first-line given its lower complication rates. Udupi and colleagues[76] compared outcomes in 40 patients who underwent GR and 39 patients who underwent RFT and found 58.9% of GR patients experienced initial pain relief, compared with 84.6% RFT patients, but this difference was not statistically significant. Rates of recurrence and the pain-free interval were also comparable.

In a review of 28 studies of surgical treatments for TN, PBC had the highest rates of durable

Table 6
Selected studies of postoperative complications after glycerol rhizotomy

Study	n	% Dysesthesia	% Anesthesia Dolorosa	% Corneal Sensory Impairment	% D plopia	% Masticatory Weakness	% Meningitis
Saini,[61] 1987	552	11.7	5.0	4.4	0	3.1	NR
Fraioli et al,[36] 1989	32	9.4	0	0	0	0	NR
Fujimaki et al,[68] 1990	122	29	2.5	NR	NR	NR	NR
Steiger,[63] 1991	122	13	NR	16	NR	4.1	0
Slettebo et al,[64] 1993	60	13.3	3.3	13.3	NR	NR	1.7
Bergenheim et al,[101] 1995	99	6.0	1.0	5.1	NR	NR	NR
Young,[62] 1998	162	3	0	4.8	NR	NR	0.6
Bender et al,[102] 2012	450	0.7	0.2	3	0.2	0	0.4

Abbreviation: NR, not recorded.
Data from Refs.[36,43,61–64,67,68]

Table 7
Selected comparative studies of percutaneous rhizotomy, microvascular decompression, and stereotactic radiosurgery

Study	Study Type	Outcome Measures	PBC	RFT	GR	MVD	SRS	Other Results
Fraioli et al,[36] 1989	Retrospective	n	n = 159	n = 533	n = 32	—	—	—
		Mean follow-up duration	3 y	6.5 y	6 y			
		% initial pain relief	89.9%	97.4%	53.1%			
		Time to recurrence	9.8%	10%	13%			
Lee et al,[103] 1997	Retrospective	n	—	n = 235	n = 36	n = 146	—	—
		Mean follow-up duration		NR	NR	5.7 y		
		% initial pain relief		92.3%	82.8%	96.5%		
		% recurrence		NR	NR	8.6%		
Henson et al,[74] 2005	Retrospective	n	—	—	n = 36	—	n = 63	—
		Mean follow-up duration			2.8 y		2.4 y	
		% initial pain relief			86%		92%	
		Time to recurrence			5 mo		8 mo	
Jellish et al,[52] 2008	Retrospective	n	n = 84	—	—	n = 80	—	Complication rate PBC 21% vs MVD 26%
		Mean follow-up duration	1.8 ± 0.3 y			2.8 ± 0.6 y		
		% initial pain relief	72%			91%		
		% recurrence	10%			11%		
		Time to recurrence (mean)	12.1 ± 3.1 mo			10.6 ± 8.5 mo		
Kouzounias et al,[75] 2010	Retrospective	n	n = 45	—	n = 101	—	—	Complication rate GR 11% vs PBC 23%
		Mean follow-up duration	NR		NR			
		% initial pain relief	85%		87%			
		Time to recurrence	21 mo		16 mo			
Udupi et al,[76] 2012	Prospective	n	—	n = 39	n = 40	—	—	—
		Mean follow-up duration		2.0 y (0.3–5)	2.5 y (0.3–4.5)			
		% initial pain relief		84.6%	58.9%			
		% recurrence		29 ± 19 mo	24 ± 15 mo			
		Time to recurrence		51.5%	39.1%			
Asplund et al,[100] 2016	Prospective	n	n = 82	—	n = 124	—	—	Corneal anesthesia and dysesthesia significantly more common after GR vs PBC
		Mean follow-up duration	5 y		5 y			
		Time to recurrence	20 mo		21 mo			

Mean follow-up duration, given in years. % initial pain relief: percentage of patients who experienced initial complete pain relief without medications. % recurrence: percentage of patients out of the total who experienced recurrence during the follow-up period. Time to recurrence: median time to pain recurrence from time of surgery, unless otherwise indicated.

Abbreviations: GR, glycerol rhizotomy; MVD, microvascular decompression; NR, not reported; PBC, percutaneous balloon compression; RFT, radiofrequency thermocoagulation; SRS, stereotactic radiosurgery.

Data from Refs.[36,41,52,74,76,100]

pain relief, but given the quality of PBC studies, no comparisons could be made with other treatment modalities. RFT was associated with high rates of pain recurrence and complications, and GR was associated with relatively lower rates of initial pain relief and shorter pain-free intervals.[22] However, the authors included only studies with at least 5 years of follow-up data. Their results also conflict with those of Lopez and colleagues,[45] who performed a systematic review of studies of percutaneous treatments and SRS and found that RFT had the highest rates of durable pain relief over 5 years. However, the 2 studies had different definitions of complete pain relief, with Tatli and colleagues including only patients who were pain-free without medications, and Lopez and colleagues, with or without medications.

Because there has been no study to demonstrate conclusively the superiority of one of the percutaneous therapies, the selection of procedure often is a reflection of the technical advantages and disadvantages of each. Advocates of PBC argue that as it is performed under general anesthesia, the patient experiences no discomfort, which can be significant with RFT.[8] In contrast, general anesthesia poses its own risk, and may not be ideal for patients with significant medical comorbidities. Although some authors argue that the lack of functional localization is a disadvantage, this technique would be well-suited for surgeons who do not see a high volume of patients with TN. As has been noted, the low rates of corneal anesthesia make the procedure well-suited for patients with isolated first division pain. The main disadvantage of the procedure is the significant bradycardia and hypotension that can result upon engagement of the foramen ovale and upon compression. Although it has been used to monitor the degree of compression, it remains a risk of the procedure.

Of the 3 percutaneous procedures, RFT is most division selective. With this, however, comes the added challenge of performing a procedure on an awake patient. Not only must the patient be able to tolerate the painful procedure, they need to participate in localization. Additionally, the procedure is associated with higher rates of anesthesia dolorosa and corneal anesthesia. Outcomes after RFT and GR are thought to be highly operator dependent compared with PBC, which is reflected in the variability across studies in the rates of pain relief. GR does not require general anesthesia and can be performed under local anesthesia with sedation, but does necessitate the patient moving from a supine to sitting position. Injection of glycerin is also more division-selective than compression. However, outcomes seem to depend on the volume of glycerin injected. In addition, the durability of the procedure has been called into question by the variability in recurrence rates across studies.[22]

MVD has often been touted as the procedure of choice for patients with TN, because it is thought to address directly the pathophysiology of the disease. In their seminal 1996 study, Barker and colleagues[79] found that the annual pain recurrence rate was 1% to 2% after MVD in the first 5 years, decreasing to less than 2% after 5 years, and less than 1% after 10 years. Although the procedure does offer high rates of durable pain relief, MVD is also associated with more severe complications.[22,52,79] Tew and colleagues[7] analyzed the outcomes of 500 patients who underwent RFT and performed a systematic review of studies of PBC, GR, and MVD. They found that RFT and MVD had the highest rates of durable pain relief, whereas GR had the highest rates of pain recurrence.

A minimally invasive treatment option for TN, SRS also has fewer operator-dependent variables. Reported of rates of initial pain relief after SRS are highly variable, from 27% to 92%.[22] Few studies directly compare outcomes of percutaneous therapies with SRS; 1 study directly compared outcomes after GR and SRS, and concluded that GR resulted in better rates of immediate pain relief, but SRS was better for durable relief.[74] Many regard SRS as most useful for patients who have recurrent TN and have undergone several other treatment modalities, seeming to provide a similar rate of initial pain relief as the initial treatment.[80] Additionally, complications are relatively rare with SRS.[45]

Although MVD may be the treatment of choice for young, healthy patients, a role for percutaneous rhizotomy remains. However, the exact patient population for which percutaneous procedures are most well-suited remains poorly defined. In a 2011 Cochrane Systematic Review of surgical interventions, the authors concluded that the quality of evidence that existed for each treatment modality was too low to provide any meaningful comparisons.[81] Comparative studies also exhibit variability in patient populations, treatment techniques, and outcomes reporting, limiting the usefulness of their conclusions. Indeed, even for MVD, only observational data were available to support the notion that it offers the highest rates of durable pain relief. Randomized, prospective trials are needed to evaluate percutaneous rhizotomy, MVD, and SRS.

Treatment Cost Effectiveness

To date, only 4 studies exist addressing the cost effectiveness of surgical interventions for

TN.[82–85] Fransen,[84] using hospital data from Belgium, compared MVD, RFT, PBC, and GK, and found comparable rates of 5- and 10-year pain recurrence. However, percutaneous procedures were more cost effective than MVD and GK. Pollock and Eller,[83] in a single-institution study of 126 patients, found that the cost per quality-adjusted pain-free year was $6342 for GR compared with $8174 for MVD. They concluded that percutaneous procedures seemed most appropriate for elderly patients with TN incompletely treated with medical therapy, but MVD was most cost effective at longer follow-up intervals.[83] Sivakanthan and colleagues,[85] using a Medicare claims database from 2011, compared MVD, SRS, and RFT. They found that although MVD was performed most frequently, RFT had a significantly lower cost per quality-adjusted life-year, at $601.64 compared with $4931.10 for MVD. However, they were unable to distinguish procedure-naïve cases from cases in which the patient had undergone prior procedures. Although the study was limited by the data available, the dramatic difference in the cost per quality-adjusted life-year underscores the importance of prospective trials comparing surgical procedures using standardized and validated outcomes measures.

Refractory or Recurrent Trigeminal Neuralgia

There is no preferred treatment for TN that recurs after an initial surgery.[86] Patients with recurrent TN are difficult to study in isolation because the majority of studies analyze do not separate these and treatment-naïve patients. There is a presumed decrement in pain relief and durability with repeat procedures; however, the relationship seems to be more complex than that.[40,87] With PBC, Kouzounias and colleagues[41] found increased complications but no decrement in pain-free interval with repeat procedures. This increased risk for complications has been shown across all treatment modalities.[22,51,79] For GR, prior RFT seems to increase the risk of postoperative sensory impairment.[43] However, the number of prior procedures does not seem to correlate with the increase in complication risk.[88]

It has been posited that repeated injections of glycerol cause intracisternal fibrosis, decreasing the effectiveness of later injections[70]; however, the largest study of repeat GR showed comparable pain-free intervals and improved rates of pain relief compared with GR in treatment-naïve patients.[67] It is possible that recurrent TN, as opposed to refractory TN, likely represents incomplete treatment or loss of treatment effect over time, whereas with refractory TN implicates a distinct pathophysiologic process that rhizotomy does not address. The variability in technique across studies likely explains the variability in outcomes, because surgeons are able to adjust the degree of compression, the volume of glycerin injected, and the location of lesion creation, among other factors, to their preference.

SUMMARY

Many elements of percutaneous rhizotomy have remained true to the techniques described by their pioneers. However, work continues to be performed to further advance and refine the methods first described by Hartel, Hakanson, Sweet, and Mullan and Lichtor. All 3 percutaneous procedures rely on Hartel's landmarks to gain access to the foramen ovale; although not considered particularly technically challenging, anatomic variants can make accessing the foramen ovale difficult and can increase the risk of complications. Much effort has been devoted to improving visualization and navigation to the foramen ovale.[89] Although fluoroscopy has been the imaging modality of choice, newer studies have demonstrated the potential usefulness of computed tomography, Dyna-computed tomography, and neuronavigation systems, especially for patients with anatomic variants that may prevent successful access with traditional means.[90–93] In 1 study of RFT, guidance with computed tomography fluoroscopy allowed for successful engagement of the foramen ovale on the first attempt, all requiring less than 40 seconds.[94] The use of neuronavigation for PBC in a series of 174 patients resulted in complete pain relief in all patients, and no complications.[92]

The success of PBC depends on adequate compression of the trigeminal ganglion, classically demonstrated by the pear shape taken on by the balloon. However, the size of the trigeminal fossa can vary significantly between patients. Goerss and colleagues[95] engineered needle cannulas of different sizes to support a range of balloon catheter sizes, from 3-F to 6-F. They described 2 cases, in which a patient failed to experience pain relief with a no. 4 Fogarty balloon who experienced durable pain relief after compression with a no. 5 Fogarty balloon. In contrast with PBC, RFT has generally been associated with higher complication rates owing to unintended damage to neurovascular structures during lesion creation. With refinement of electrodes to allow for small lesions, complication rates decreased but remained relatively high compared with PBC and GR. The size of the lesion not only depends on the size of the electrode tip and the electrode diameter, but also the duration of thermocoagulation and the temperature achieved in the tissue. Karol and colleagues[96] designed a quadripolar electrode able to create lesions one-third the size attained by that of a standard Tew electrode. Additional clinical studies are required to investigate the potential benefit of these electrodes. Pulsed radiofrequency current, in which the current is delivered in bursts, allows the heat to dissipate and maintains the tissue at a lower temperature. The technique has been used successfully to treat spinal pain, and early reports of its use in patients with TN have been promising. Erdine and colleagues used pulsed radiofrequency current to treat 5 patients; 3 (60%) experienced durable pain relief and no neurologic complications were observed.[97,98]

Percutaneous rhizotomy, in all its forms, offers pain relief for TN that is immediate with varying durability and a generally favorable side effect profile. However, treatment selection remains an inexact science in the absence of high quality outcomes data. In addition to incorporating these technical advances, future studies must overcome the patient heterogeneity, procedural variation, and nonstandard outcomes that limit interpretation of the existing literature.

ACKNOWLEDGMENTS

Joanna Y. Wang, BA, Department of Neurosurgery, Johns Hopkins University School of Medicine, Baltimore, MD contributed to the writing of this article.

REFERENCES

1. Cheng JS, Lim DA, Chang EF, et al. A review of percutaneous treatments for trigeminal neuralgia. Neurosurgery 2014;10(Suppl 1):25–33 [discussion: 33].
2. Wang DD, Ouyang D, Englot DJ, et al. Trends in surgical treatment for trigeminal neuralgia in the United States of America from 1988 to 2008. J Clin Neurosci 2013;20(11):1538–45.
3. Cole CD, Liu JK, Apfelbaum RI. Historical perspectives on the diagnosis and treatment of trigeminal neuralgia. Neurosurg Focus 2005;18(5):E4.
4. Skirving DJ, Dan NG. A 20-year review of percutaneous balloon compression of the trigeminal ganglion. J Neurosurg 2001;94(6):913–7.
5. Brown JA. Percutaneous balloon compression for trigeminal neuralgia. Clin Neurosurg 2009;56:73–8.
6. Sweet WH, Wepsic JG. Controlled thermocoagulation of trigeminal ganglion and rootlets for differential destruction of pain fibers. 1. Trigeminal neuralgia. J Neurosurg 1974;40(2):143–56.
7. Tew JM, Morgan CJ, Grande AW. Percutaneous rhizotomy in the treatment of intractable facial pain (trigeminal, glossopharyngeal, and vagal nerves). In: Schmidek HH, Sweet WH, editors. Operative neurosurgical techniques: indications, methods and results. 3 edition. Philadelphia: WB Saunders; 1996. p. 1409–18.
8. Nugent GR. Radiofrequency treatment of trigeminal neuralgia using a cordotomy-type electrode. A method. Neurosurg Clin N Am 1997;8(1): 41–52.
9. Håkanson S. Stereotactic radiosurgery in trigeminal neuralgia. New York: Gustav Fischer Verlag; 1979.
10. Lunsford LD, Bennett MH. Percutaneous retrogasserian glycerol rhizotomy for tic douloureux: Part 1. Technique and results in 112 patients. Neurosurgery 1984;14(4):424–30.
11. Bennett MH, Lunsford LD. Percutaneous retrogasserian glycerol rhizotomy for tic douloureux: Part 2. Results and implications of trigeminal evoked potential studies. Neurosurgery 1984; 14(4):431–5.
12. Dulhunty AF, Gage PW. Differential effects of glycerol treatment on membrane capacity and excitation-contraction coupling in toad sartorius fibres. J Physiol 1973;234(2):373–408.
13. King JS, Jewett DL, Sundberg HR. Differential blockade of cat dorsal root C fibers by various chloride solutions. J Neurosurg 1972;36(5): 569–83.
14. Linderoth B, Lind G. Retrogasserian glycerol rhizolysis in trigeminal neuralgia. In: Quiñones-Hinojosa A, editor. Schmidek and Sweet's Operative neurosurgical techniques. Philadelphia: Saunders; 2012. p. 1393–408.
15. Robertson JD. Structural alterations in nerve fibers produced by hypotonic and hypertonic solutions. J Biophys Biochem Cytol 1958;4(4):349–64.
16. Pal HK, Dinda AK, Roy S, et al. Acute effect of anhydrous glycerol on peripheral nerve: an experimental study. Br J Neurosurg 1989;3(4): 463–9.
17. Taarnhoj P. Decompression of the trigeminal root and the posterior part of the ganglion as treatment in trigeminal neuralgia; preliminary communication. J Neurosurg 1952;9(3):288–90.
18. Shelden CH, Pudenz RH, Freshwater DB, et al. Compression rather than decompression for trigeminal neuralgia. J Neurosurg 1955;12(2):123–6.
19. Mullan S, Lichtor T. Percutaneous microcompression of the trigeminal ganglion for trigeminal neuralgia. J Neurosurg 1983;59(6):1007–12.
20. Brown JA, Hoeflinger B, Long PB, et al. Axon and ganglion cell injury in rabbits after percutaneous trigeminal balloon compression. Neurosurgery 1996; 38(5):993–1003 [discussion: 1003–4].

21. Eller JL, Raslan AM, Burchiel KJ. Trigeminal neuralgia: definition and classification. Neurosurg Focus 2005;18(5):E3.
22. Tatli M, Satici O, Kanpolat Y, et al. Various surgical modalities for trigeminal neuralgia: literature study of respective long-term outcomes. Acta Neurochir (Wien) 2008;150(3):243–55.
23. Gronseth G, Cruccu G, Alksne J, et al. Practice parameter: the diagnostic evaluation and treatment of trigeminal neuralgia (an evidence-based review) - report of the quality standards subcommittee of the American Academy of and the European Federation of Neurological Societies. Neurology 2008;71(15):1183–90.
24. Dalessio DJ. Trigeminal neuralgia. A practical approach to treatment. Drugs 1982;24(3):248–55.
25. North RB, Kidd DH, Piantadosi S, et al. Percutaneous retrogasserian glycerol rhizotomy. Predictors of success and failure in treatment of trigeminal neuralgia. J Neurosurg 1990;72(6):851–6.
26. Zakrzewska JM, Jassim S, Bulman JS. A prospective, longitudinal study on patients with trigeminal neuralgia who underwent radiofrequency thermocoagulation of the gasserian ganglion. Pain 1999;79(1):51–8.
27. O'Connor AB, Schwid SR, Herrmann DN, et al. Pain associated with multiple sclerosis: systematic review and proposed classification. Pain 2008; 137(1):96–111.
28. Mohammad-Mohammadi A, Recinos PF, Lee JH, et al. Surgical outcomes of trigeminal neuralgia in patients with multiple sclerosis. Neurosurgery 2013;73(6):941–50 [discussion: 950].
29. Kondziolka D, Lunsford LD, Bissonette DJ. Long-term results after glycerol rhizotomy for multiple sclerosis-related trigeminal neuralgia. Can J Neurol Sci 1994;21(2):137–40.
30. Cheng JS, Sanchez-Mejia RO, Limbo M, et al. Management of medically refractory trigeminal neuralgia in patients with multiple sclerosis. Neurosurg Focus 2005;18(5):e13.
31. Pickett GE, Bisnaire D, Ferguson GG. Percutaneous retrogasserian glycerol rhizotomy in the treatment of tic douloureux associated with multiple sclerosis. Neurosurgery 2005;56(3):537–45 [discussion: 537–45].
32. Sandell T, Eide PK. The effect of microvascular decompression in patients with multiple sclerosis and trigeminal neuralgia. Neurosurgery 2010; 67(3):749–53 [discussion: 753–44].
33. Abdennebi B, Mahfouf L, Nedjahi T. Long-term results of percutaneous compression of the gasserian ganglion in trigeminal neuralgia (series of 200 patients). Stereotact Funct Neurosurg 1997;68(1–4 Pt 1):190–5.
34. Brown JA, Pilitsis JG. Percutaneous balloon compression for the treatment of trigeminal neuralgia: results in 56 patients based on balloon compression pressure monitoring. Neurosurg Focus 2005;18(5):E10.
35. Lichtor T, Mullan JF. A 10-year follow-up review of percutaneous microcompression of the trigeminal ganglion. J Neurosurg 1990;72(1):49–54.
36. Fraioli B, Esposito V, Guidetti B, et al. Treatment of trigeminal neuralgia by thermocoagulation, glycerolization, and percutaneous compression of the gasserian ganglion and/or retrogasserian rootlets: long-term results and therapeutic protocol. Neurosurgery 1989;24(2):239–45.
37. Lobato RD, Rivas JJ, Sarabia R, et al. Percutaneous microcompression of the gasserian ganglion for trigeminal neuralgia. J Neurosurg 1990;72(4): 546–53.
38. Brown JA, McDaniel MD, Weaver MT. Percutaneous trigeminal nerve compression for treatment of trigeminal neuralgia: results in 50 patients. Neurosurgery 1993;32(4):570–3.
39. Correa CF, Teixeira MJ. Balloon compression of the gasserian ganglion for the treatment of trigeminal neuralgia. Stereotact Funct Neurosurg 1998;71(2): 83–9.
40. Omeis I, Smith D, Kim S, et al. Percutaneous balloon compression for the treatment of recurrent trigeminal neuralgia: long-term outcome in 29 patients. Stereotact Funct Neurosurg 2008;86(4):259–65.
41. Kouzounias K, Schechtmann G, Lind G, et al. Factors that influence outcome of percutaneous balloon compression in the treatment of trigeminal neuralgia. Neurosurgery 2010;67(4):925–34 [discussion: 934].
42. Chen JF, Tu PH, Lee ST. Long-term follow-up of patients treated with percutaneous balloon compression for trigeminal neuralgia in Taiwan. World Neurosurg 2011;76(6):586–91.
43. Bergenheim AT, Asplund P, Linderoth B. Percutaneous retrogasserian balloon compression for trigeminal neuralgia: review of critical technical details and outcomes. World Neurosurg 2013; 79(2):359–68.
44. Abdennebi B, Guenane L. Technical considerations and outcome assessment in retrogasserian balloon compression for treatment of trigeminal neuralgia. Series of 901 patients. Surg Neurol Int 2014;5:118.
45. Lopez BC, Hamlyn PJ, Zakrzewska JM. Systematic review of ablative neurosurgical techniques for the treatment of trigeminal neuralgia. Neurosurgery 2004;54(4):973–82 [discussion: 982–3].
46. Chroni E, Constantoyannis C, Prasoulis I, et al. Masseter muscle function after percutaneous balloon compression of trigeminal ganglion for the treatment of trigeminal neuralgia: a neurophysiological follow-up study. Clin Neurophysiol 2011; 122(2):410–3.

47. de Siqueira SR, da Nobrega JC, de Siqueira JT, et al. Frequency of postoperative complications after balloon compression for idiopathic trigeminal neuralgia: prospective study. Oral Surg Oral Med Oral Pathol Oral Radiol Endod 2006;102(5):e39–45.
48. Agazzi S, Chang S, Drucker MD, et al. Sudden blindness as a complication of percutaneous trigeminal procedures: mechanism analysis and prevention. J Neurosurg 2009;110(4):638–41.
49. Liu HB, Ma Y, Zou JJ, et al. Percutaneous microballoon compression for trigeminal neuralgia. Chin Med J 2007;120(3):228–30.
50. Asplund P, Linderoth B, Bergenheim AT. The predictive power of balloon shape and change of sensory functions on outcome of percutaneous balloon compression for trigeminal neuralgia. J Neurosurg 2010;113(3):498–507.
51. Lee ST, Chen JF. Percutaneous trigeminal ganglion balloon compression for treatment of trigeminal neuralgia, part II: results related to compression duration. Surg Neurol 2003;60(2):149–53 [discussion: 153–4].
52. Jellish WS, Benedict W, Owen K, et al. Perioperative and long-term operative outcomes after surgery for trigeminal neuralgia: microvascular decompression vs percutaneous balloon ablation. Head Face Med 2008;4:11.
53. Frank F, Fabrizi AP. Percutaneous surgical treatment of trigeminal neuralgia. Acta Neurochir (Wien) 1989;97(3–4):128–30.
54. Broggi G, Franzini A, Lasio G, et al. Long-term results of percutaneous retrogasserian thermorhizotomy for "essential" trigeminal neuralgia: considerations in 1000 consecutive patients. Neurosurgery 1990; 26(5):783–6 [discussion: 786–7].
55. Scrivani SJ, Keith DA, Mathews ES, et al. Percutaneous stereotactic differential radiofrequency thermal rhizotomy for the treatment of trigeminal neuralgia. J Oral Maxillofac Surg 1999;57(2): 104–11 [discussion: 111–2].
56. Tronnier VM, Rasche D, Hamer J, et al. Treatment of idiopathic trigeminal neuralgia: comparison of long-term outcome after radiofrequency rhizotomy and microvascular decompression. Neurosurgery 2001;48(6):1261–7 [discussion: 1267–8].
57. Kanpolat Y, Savas A, Bekar A, et al. Percutaneous controlled radiofrequency trigeminal rhizotomy for the treatment of idiopathic trigeminal neuralgia: 25-year experience with 1,600 patients. Neurosurgery 2001;48(3):524–32 [discussion: 532–4].
58. Taha JM, Tew JM Jr. Comparison of surgical treatments for trigeminal neuralgia: reevaluation of radiofrequency rhizotomy. Neurosurgery 1996;38(5): 865–71.
59. Rath GP, Dash HH, Bithal PK, et al. Intracranial hemorrhage after percutaneous radiofrequency trigeminal rhizotomy. Pain Pract 2009;9(1):82–4.
60. Kosugi S, Shiotani M, Otsuka Y, et al. Long-term outcomes of percutaneous radiofrequency thermocoagulation of gasserian ganglion for 2nd- and multiple-division trigeminal neuralgia. Pain Pract 2015;15(3):223–8.
61. Saini SS. Reterogasserian anhydrous glycerol injection therapy in trigeminal neuralgia: observations in 552 patients. J Neurol Neurosurg Psychiatry 1987;50(11):1536–8.
62. Young RF. Glycerol rhizolysis for treatment of trigeminal neuralgia. J Neurosurg 1988;69(1): 39–45.
63. Steiger HJ. Prognostic factors in the treatment of trigeminal neuralgia. Analysis of a differential therapeutic approach. Acta Neurochir (Wien) 1991; 113(1–2):11–7.
64. Slettebo H, Hirschberg H, Lindegaard KF. Long-term results after percutaneous retrogasserian glycerol rhizotomy in patients with trigeminal neuralgia. Acta Neurochir (Wien) 1993;122(3–4):231–5.
65. Erdem E, Alkan A. Peripheral glycerol injections in the treatment of idiopathic trigeminal neuralgia: retrospective analysis of 157 cases. J Oral Maxillofac Surg 2001;59(10):1176–80.
66. Pollock BE. Percutaneous retrogasserian glycerol rhizotomy for patients with idiopathic trigeminal neuralgia: a prospective analysis of factors related to pain relief. J Neurosurg 2005;102(2):223–8.
67. Bender MT, Pradilla G, Batra S, et al. Glycerol rhizotomy and radiofrequency thermocoagulation for trigeminal neuralgia in multiple sclerosis. J Neurosurg 2013;118(2):329–36.
68. Fujimaki T, Fukushima T, Miyazaki S. Percutaneous retrogasserian glycerol injection in the management of trigeminal neuralgia: long-term follow-up results. J Neurosurg 1990;73(2):212–6.
69. Jagia M, Bithal PK, Dash HH, et al. Effect of cerebrospinal fluid return on success rate of percutaneous retrogasserian glycerol rhizotomy. Reg Anesth Pain Med 2004;29(6):592–5.
70. Rappaport ZH, Gomori JM. Recurrent trigeminal cistern glycerol injections for tic douloureux. Acta Neurochir (Wien) 1988;90(1–2):31–4.
71. Dieckmann G, Bockermann V, Heyer C, et al. Five-and-a-half years' experience with percutaneous retrogasserian glycerol rhizotomy in treatment of trigeminal neuralgia. Appl Neurophysiol 1987; 50(1–6):401–13.
72. Pandia MP, Dash HH, Bithal PK, et al. Does egress of cerebrospinal fluid during percutaneous retrogasserian glycerol rhizotomy influence long term pain relief? Reg Anesth Pain Med 2008;33(3):222–6.
73. Rogers CL, Shetter AG, Fiedler JA, et al. Gamma knife radiosurgery for trigeminal neuralgia: the initial experience of The Barrow Neurological Institute. Int J Radiat Oncol Biol Phys 2000;47(4):1013–9.

74. Henson CF, Goldman HW, Rosenwasser RH, et al. Glycerol rhizotomy versus gamma knife radiosurgery for the treatment of trigeminal neuralgia: an analysis of patients treated at one institution. Int J Radiat Oncol Biol Phys 2005;63(1):82–90.
75. Kouzounias K, Lind G, Schechtmann G, et al. Comparison of percutaneous balloon compression and glycerol rhizotomy for the treatment of trigeminal neuralgia. J Neurosurg 2010;113(3): 486–92.
76. Udupi BP, Chouhan RS, Dash HH, et al. Comparative evaluation of percutaneous retrogasserian glycerol rhizolysis and radiofrequency thermocoagulation techniques in the management of trigeminal neuralgia. Neurosurgery 2012;70(2):407–12 [discussion: 412–3].
77. Lee KH, Chang JW, Park YG, et al. Microvascular decompression and percutaneous rhizotomy in trigeminal neuralgia. Stereotact Funct Neurosurg 1997;68(1–4 Pt 1):196–9.
78. Haridas A, Mathewson C, Eljamel S. Long-term results of 405 refractory trigeminal neuralgia surgeries in 256 patients. Zentralbl Neurochir 2008; 69(4):170–4.
79. Barker FG 2nd, Jannetta PJ, Bissonette DJ, et al. The long-term outcome of microvascular decompression for trigeminal neuralgia. N Engl J Med 1996;334(17):1077–83.
80. Hasegawa T, Kondziolka D, Spiro R, et al. Repeat radiosurgery for refractory trigeminal neuralgia. Neurosurgery 2002;50(3):494–500 [discussion 500–2].
81. Zakrzewska JM, Akram H. Neurosurgical interventions for the treatment of classical trigeminal neuralgia. Cochrane Database Syst Rev 2011;(9):CD007312.
82. Holland M, Noeller J, Buatti J, et al. The cost-effectiveness of surgery for trigeminal neuralgia in surgically naive patients: a retrospective study. Clin Neurol Neurosurg 2015;137:34–7.
83. Pollock BE, Ecker RD. A prospective cost-effectiveness study of trigeminal neuralgia surgery. Clin J Pain 2005;21(4):317–22.
84. Fransen P. Cost-effectiveness in the surgical treatments for trigeminal neuralgia. Acta Neurol Belg 2012;112(3):245–7.
85. Sivakanthan S, Van Gompel JJ, Alikhani P, et al. Surgical management of trigeminal neuralgia: use and cost-effectiveness from an analysis of the Medicare Claims Database. Neurosurgery 2014; 75(3):220–6 [discussion: 225–6].
86. Pollock BE, Stein KJ. Surgical management of trigeminal neuralgia patients with recurrent or persistent pain despite three or more prior operations. World Neurosurg 2010;73(5):523–8.
87. Montano N, Papacci F, Cioni B, et al. What is the best treatment of drug-resistant trigeminal neuralgia in patients affected by multiple sclerosis? A literature analysis of surgical procedures. Clin Neurol Neurosurg 2013;115(5):567–72.
88. Harries AM, Mitchell RD. Percutaneous glycerol rhizotomy for trigeminal neuralgia: safety and efficacy of repeat procedures. Br J Neurosurg 2011;25(2): 268–72.
89. Peris-Celda M, Graziano F, Russo V, et al. Foramen ovale puncture, lesioning accuracy, and avoiding complications: microsurgical anatomy study with clinical implications. J Neurosurg 2013;119(5): 1176–93.
90. Huo X, Sun X, Zhang Z, et al. Dyna-CT-assisted percutaneous microballoon compression for trigeminal neuralgia. J Neurointerv Surg 2014;6(7):521–6.
91. Aydoseli A, Akcakaya MO, Aras Y, et al. Neuronavigation-assisted percutaneous balloon compression for the treatment of trigeminal neuralgia: the technique and short-term clinical results. Br J Neurosurg 2015;29(4):552–8.
92. Georgiopoulos M, Ellul J, Chroni E, et al. Minimizing technical failure of percutaneous balloon compression for trigeminal neuralgia using neuronavigation. ISRN Neurol 2014;2014:630418.
93. Xu SJ, Zhang WH, Chen T, et al. Neuronavigator-guided percutaneous radiofrequency thermocoagulation in the treatment of intractable trigeminal neuralgia. Chin Med J 2006;119(18):1528–35.
94. Gusmao S, Oliveira M, Tazinaffo U, et al. Percutaneous trigeminal nerve radiofrequency rhizotomy guided by computerized tomography fluoroscopy. Technical note. J Neurosurg 2003;99(4):785–6.
95. Goerss SJ, Atkinson JL, Kallmes DF. Variable size percutaneous balloon compression of the gasserian ganglion for trigeminal neuralgia. Surg Neurol 2009;71(3):388–90 [discussion: 391].
96. Karol EA, Karol MN. A multiarray electrode mapping method for percutaneous thermocoagulation as treatment of trigeminal neuralgia. Technical note on a series of 178 consecutive procedures. Surg Neurol 2009;71(1):11–7 [discussion: 17–8].
97. Van Zundert J, Brabant S, Van de Kelft E, et al. Pulsed radiofrequency treatment of the Gasserian ganglion in patients with idiopathic trigeminal neuralgia. Pain 2003;104(3):449–52.
98. Erdine S, Ozyalcin NS, Cimen A, et al. Comparison of pulsed radiofrequency with conventional radiofrequency in the treatment of idiopathic trigeminal neuralgia. Eur J Pain 2007;11(3):309–13.
99. Brown JA, Gouda JJ. Percutaneous balloon compression of the trigeminal nerve. Neurosurg Clin N Am 1997;8(1):53–62.
100. Asplund P, Blomstedt P, Bergenheim AT. Percutaneous balloon compression vs percutaneous retrogasserian glycerol rhizotomy for the primary treatment of trigeminal neuralgia. Neurosurgery 2016;78(3):421–8.

101. Bergenheim AT, Hariz MI. Influence of previous treatment on outcome after glycerol rhizotomy for trigeminal neuralgia. Neurosurgery 1995;36(2): 303–9.
102. Bender M, Pradilla G, Batra S, et al. Effectiveness of repeat glycerol rhizotomy in treating recurrent trigeminal neuralgia. Neurosurgery 2012;70(5): 1125–33.
103. Lee KH, Chang JW, Park YG, et al. Microvascular decompression and percutaneous rhizotomy in trigeminal neuralgia. Stereotact Funct Neurosurg 1997;68(1-4 Pt 1):196–9.

Gamma Knife Surgery in Trigeminal Neuralgia

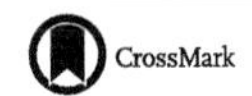

Amparo Wolf, MD, PhD[a], Douglas Kondziolka, MD, MSc, FRCSC[b,*]

KEYWORDS

• Trigeminal neuralgia • Gamma knife surgery • Stereotactic radiosurgery • Facial pain

KEY POINTS

- Gamma Knife surgery (GKS) represents a safe, effective, and relatively durable noninvasive treatment option for patients with trigeminal neuralgia (TN) and recurrent TN.
- Predictors of durability of GKS in TN include type I TN, post-GKS Barrow Neurological Institute score, and the presence of post Gamma Knife facial numbness.
- GKS performed earlier in the course of disease and as an initial procedure may result in a shorter interval to pain relief and longer pain-free intervals.
- Patients report significant improvements in quality of life after GKS for TN.

INTRODUCTION

Since the initial report by Dr Leksell in 1971[1] and early reports from the 1990s,[2–4] the role of Gamma Knife surgery (GKS) in patients with intractable trigeminal neuralgia (TN) has been growing exponentially. GKS is a minimally invasive surgical approach for TN, within the armamentarium of a neurosurgeon, along with more invasive procedures including percutaneous ablative procedures (thermal rhizotomy, glycerol rhizotomy, or balloon microcompression) and craniotomy for microvascular decompression (MVD).

To date, greater than 450 articles have been published looking at the safety and effectiveness of GKS in the treatment of TN or recurrent TN. This report summarizes the literature on the effectiveness of GKS for pain relief, the latency until pain relief, the durability of pain relief, and predictors of its success.

EFFECTIVENESS OF GAMMA KNIFE SURGERY FOR IDIOPATHIC TRIGEMINAL NEURALGIA

There are 4 key studies published within the last 5 years that report on the effectiveness of GKS in a large population of type I TN patients and with long-term outcomes (**Table 1**). By 1 year's time, 75% to 90% of patients will have obtained pain relief, defined as Barrow Neurological Institute (BNI) grades I to IIIB.[5–8] Achieving BNI I may prove more challenging because of the reluctance of some patients to discontinue their medication for fear of the pain recurring. **Fig. 1** depicts a treatment plan of a 54 year old woman with right-sided TN who underwent GKS to the right trigeminal nerve at a maximum dose of 80 Gy.

Although there are no randomized control studies directly comparing GKS to other surgical procedures for TN, the pain relief rates in the studies listed in **Table 1** are similar to those reported for MVD.[9,10] A select few studies have directly compared GKS to either MVD or rhizotomy.[11–13] Similar improvements in pain were reported between rhizotomy and GKS,[11] however, with faster onset of pain relief and higher morbidities after rhizotomy. Collectively, MVD offers higher rates of longer-term, pain-free outcomes, compared with GKS,[12,13] however, at a higher complication rate, including cerebrospinal fluid leak, cranial neuropathies, wound infection, deep vein thrombosis, and pulmonary embolism.

Disclosure Statement: The authors have nothing to disclose.

[a] Department of Neurosurgery, NYU Langone Medical Center, 530 First Avenue, Suite 8R, New York, NY 10016, USA; [b] Department of Neurosurgery, Center for Advanced Radiosurgery, NYU Langone Medical Center, 530 First Avenue, Suite 8R, New York, NY 10016, USA
* Corresponding author.
E-mail address: douglas.kondziolka@nyumc.org

Neurosurg Clin N Am 27 (2016) 297–304
http://dx.doi.org/10.1016/j.nec.2016.02.006
1042-3680/16/$ – see front matter

Table 1
Selected large series of Gamma Knife radiosurgery for type I trigeminal neuralgia with long-term outcomes

Study	N	Median Maximum Dose (Gy)	Median Follow-Up (mo)	Pain Free (%)	Recurrence (%)	Median Time to Recurrence	Sensory Dysfunction (%)
Regis et al,[5] 2015	497	85	43.8	*BNI1:* 6 mo: 91.8 5 y: 64.9	34.4	24	14.5
Lucas et al,[6] 2014	446	90	21.2	*BNI1-3B:* 1 y: 84.5 5 y: 46.9 *BNI1:* 1 y: 62.9 5 y: 22.0	45.1	55.2	42.0
Marshall et al,[7] 2012	448	88 (mean)	20.9	**BNI1-3B:* 1 y: ~75 5 y: ~50	40.0	58.4	42.0
Kondziolka et al,[8] 2010	503	80	24.0	*BNI1-3B:* 1 y: 80.0 5 y: 46.0	42.9	48	10.5

* Estimated from graph of Kaplan-Meier curve in Marshall et al, 2012.
Data from Refs.[5–8]

LATENCY UNTIL PAIN RELIEF AFTER GAMMA KNIFE SURGERY

Multiple studies have confirmed a median latency period of 1 to 2 months before the onset of pain relief after GKS.[2,14,15] In the largest study of 503 patients, Kondziolka and colleagues[8] found that 89% of patients responded to treatment at a median of 1 month, and total pain relief was achieved at a median of 5 months. Predictors of faster pain relief included GKS as the initial surgical procedure, within 3 years of pain onset.[8]

In patients with severe pain that is intractable to all medical therapies, a lengthy delay between treatment and pain relief may be intolerable, and thus, other surgical treatments that provide immediate pain relief may be desirable, such as glycerol rhizotomy, with which pain relief is felt to be immediate within days.[11]

DURABILITY OF PAIN RELIEF WITH GAMMA KNIFE SURGERY AND PREDICTORS OF SUCCESS

From **Table 1**, by 5 years after GKS, 46% to 65% of type 1 TN patients remain with well-controlled pain (BNI I–IIIb). According to a multivariate analysis performed by the group at Wake Forest, predictors of the durability of GKS in TN patients include the presenting Burchiel pain type, the post-GKS BNI score, and the presence of post-GKS facial numbness.[6] Post-GKS numbness has been identified as a major predictor of the success in multiple series.[7,8,16] Another report found that patients who responded to GKS within the first 3 weeks predicted a longer duration of complete pain relief.[17] Multiple studies have identified that type 2 TN patients are at greater risk of pain relapse after GKS.[6,18] Nevertheless, patients with multiple sclerosis (or symptomatic TN based on Burchiel's classification) may benefit from GKS with response rates reported between 57% and 97%[18–20] and long-term pain relief outcomes potentially similar to patients with idiopathic TN.[19]

One study suggested that neurovascular conflict resulted in improved outcomes after GKS.[21] However, the underlying pathophysiology of TN and relationship to microvascular compression remain to be elucidated. TN appears to be a complex disorder with subtypes that may manifest at different ages, such that younger patients are less likely to have neurovascular conflict.[22] Whether different subtypes of idiopathic TN may respond better to Stereotactic radiosurgery (SRS) is unknown at this time.

SIDE EFFECTS OF GAMMA KNIFE SURGERY FOR TRIGEMINAL NEURALGIA

The most common side effect reported is trigeminal nerve sensory disturbance, and this appears to be dose-dependent. Reported rates of persistent sensory dysfunction range from 10% to 42%

see **Table 1**). Matsuda and colleagues[23] followed patients every 3 months after GKS and assessed trigeminal nerve dysfunction using the Barrow Neurological Institute Numbness scale (BNI-N). They reported trigeminal nerve dysfunction of 49% at 3 months, which reduced to 41.3% at a median time of 37 months; 25% were categorized as BNI-N Score II, 12.5% as BNI-N Score III, and 3.8% as BNI-N Score IV.[23] This trend of decreasing incidence of sensory dysfunction over time fits with many prior reports.[24,25] The vast majority of patients often do not find the post-GKS numbness bothersome or disabling.[5] However, a trigeminal sensory deficit may rarely be associated with a reduced corneal reflex, and thus, patients may be at risk of a corneal injury.

The placement of the target isocenter may be associated with the development of sensory dysfunction. Rates of numbness were reported as low as 10% at 12 months after radiosurgery, when placing the target in the anterior cisternal portion of the nerve.[24] However, in another study

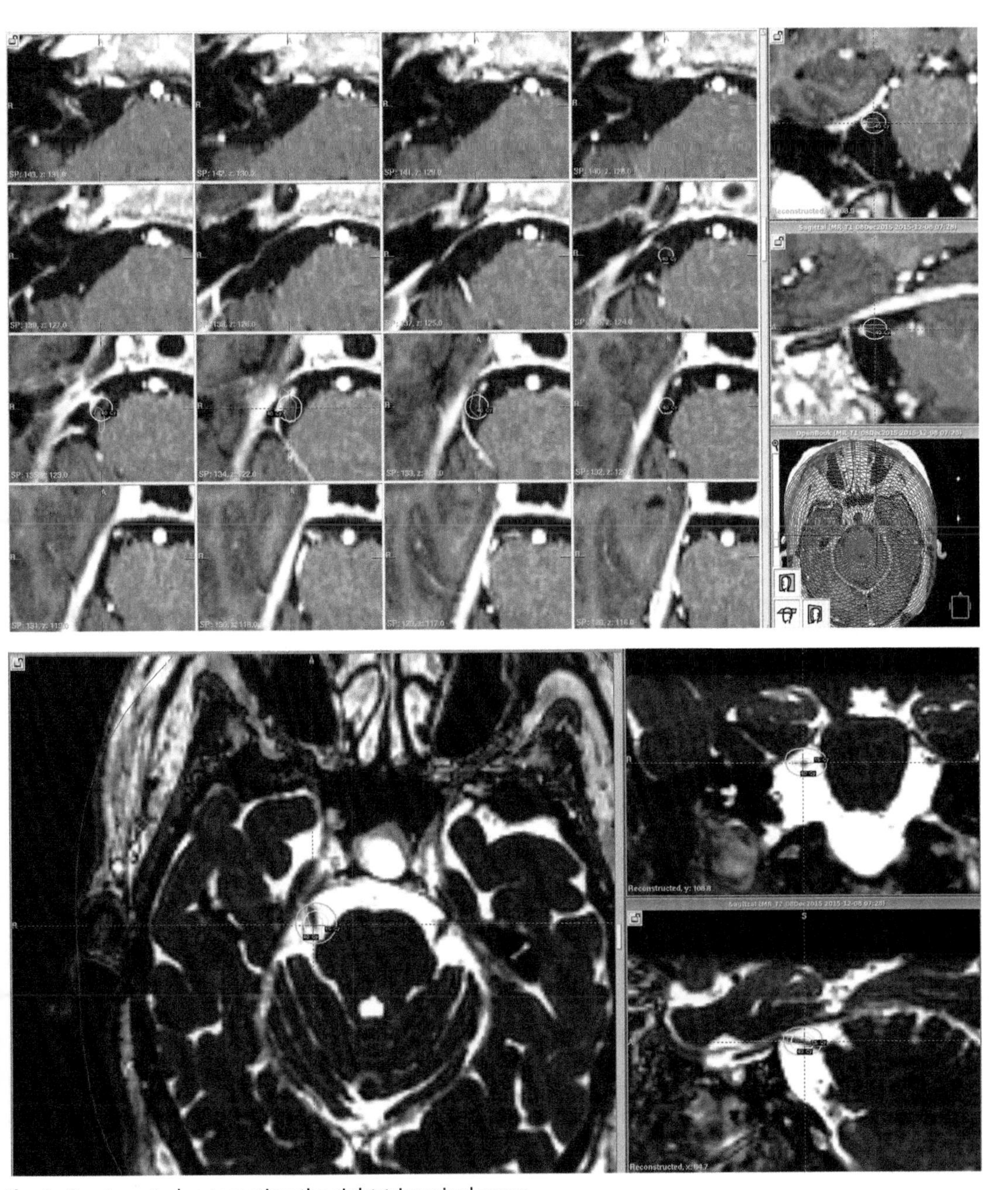

Fig. 1. Treatment plan targeting the right trigeminal nerve.

also targeting the anterior cisternal portion of the trigeminal nerve, their rates for sensory deficit was 34%.[26] However, their radiation dose was higher. A radiation dose of 90 Gy to the trigeminal nerve and higher doses to the brainstem may be associated with increased incidence of bothersome sensory dysfunction and/or numbness.[27,28]

In addition to target location and radiation dose, other factors that may predispose to post-GKS sensory neuropathy are the dose to the brainstem and the length of nerve included within the target zone. In a prospective randomized study comparing 1 or 2 isocenters in patients with TN who underwent GKS, longer nerve irradiation with 2 isocenters resulted in a higher complication rate with no significant difference in effectiveness.[29]

As noted in one report using Cyberknife for TN, other complications may occur, although infrequently, including masticator weakness, diplopia, and decreased hearing.[30] In this study, the investigators identified that higher radiation doses and treating longer segments of the nerve resulted in an increased rate of complications.

THE ROLE OF REPEAT GAMMA KNIFE SURGERY FOR TRIGEMINAL NEURALGIA

The effectiveness of repeat GKS has been investigated in numerous retrospective, single-institution, small sample studies[31] (see Ref.[31] for systematic review). Only 2 studies to date have looked at outcomes of repeat SRS in more than 100 patients (**Table 2**). In a recent systematic analysis reviewing 20 published studies on repeat GKS in TN, the median time between first and second GKS was 17 months.[31] Outcomes after second GKS were variable, with a median rate of pain cessation of 88% (60%–100%) after second GKS and a median hypesthesia rate of 33% (11%–80%). Park and colleagues[32] reviewed outcomes of 119 patients and identified predictors of success for recurrent TN after having failed initial GKS. They found that development of sensory loss and recurrent pain in a reduced facial distribution compared with initial GKS predicted long-term pain control. These results were corroborated by another study looking at predictors of success for repeat SRS, which included facial numbness after the first GKS and a positive pain response.[33]

Potentially even a third GKS for TN may be performed. One study reported on 17 patients with refractory TN undergoing a third GKS.[34] No patients experienced additional sensory disturbances. Seventy-six percent of patients had complete pain relief or improved pain, whereas 24% had recurrence of pain at a mean interval of 19.1 months. Overall, these results suggest that a third GKS procedure may provide pain relief with a low risk of complications and may be worthwhile to pursue in patients who are not candidates for microsurgical or percutaneous procedures.[34]

IS THERE AN OPTIMAL TIME TO UNDERGO GAMMA KNIFE SURGERY FOR TRIGEMINAL NEURALGIA?

The pain-free incidence and latency to pain relief post-GKS in TN patients with a history of previous surgeries (MVD or rhizotomy) are

Table 2
Selected large series of repeat Gamma Knife radiosurgery for trigeminal neuralgia

Study	N	Median Maximum Dose 2nd Procedure (Gy)	Median Follow-Up (mo)	Pain Free (%)	Recurrence (%)	Median Time to Recurrence	Sensory Dysfunction (%)
Park et al,[32] 2012	119	70	48	*BNI I-IIIB:* 1 y: 87.8 5 y: 44.2	34	26	21
Helis et al,[33] 2015	125	80	27.1	*BNI I-IIIB:* 1 y: 78 5 y: 49 *BNI I:* 1 y: 63.0 5 y: 37.0	20	20	70

Data from Park KJ, Kondziolka D, Berkowitz O, et al. Repeat gamma knife radiosurgery for trigeminal neuralgia. Neurosurgery 2012;70(2):295–305; [discussion: 305]; and Helis CA, Lucas JT, Bourland JD, et al. Repeat radiosurgery for trigeminal neuralgia. Neurosurgery 2015;77(5):755–61.

generally reduced.[27,35] Longhi and colleagues[35] reported that for patients who had no previous surgery, more than 70% had an excellent response, in contrast to 40% in patients with previous surgical treatment. Whether performing GKS earlier is of any benefit was recently addressed in a retrospective study by the Pittsburgh group. They looked at 121 patients with refractory TN and found that shorter interval to pain relief, longer pain-free intervals, and longer time off medications were achieved if treated within 3 years of diagnosis of TN and as an initial surgical procedure.[17]

QUALITY OF LIFE IN PATIENTS WITH TRIGEMINAL NEURALGIA

Several studies have examined the impact of GKS for TN on patient-rated satisfaction and quality of life (QOL). The key factors impacting QOL include pain relief, trigeminal nerve dysfunction, and medication side effects. Using the Epilepsy Surgery

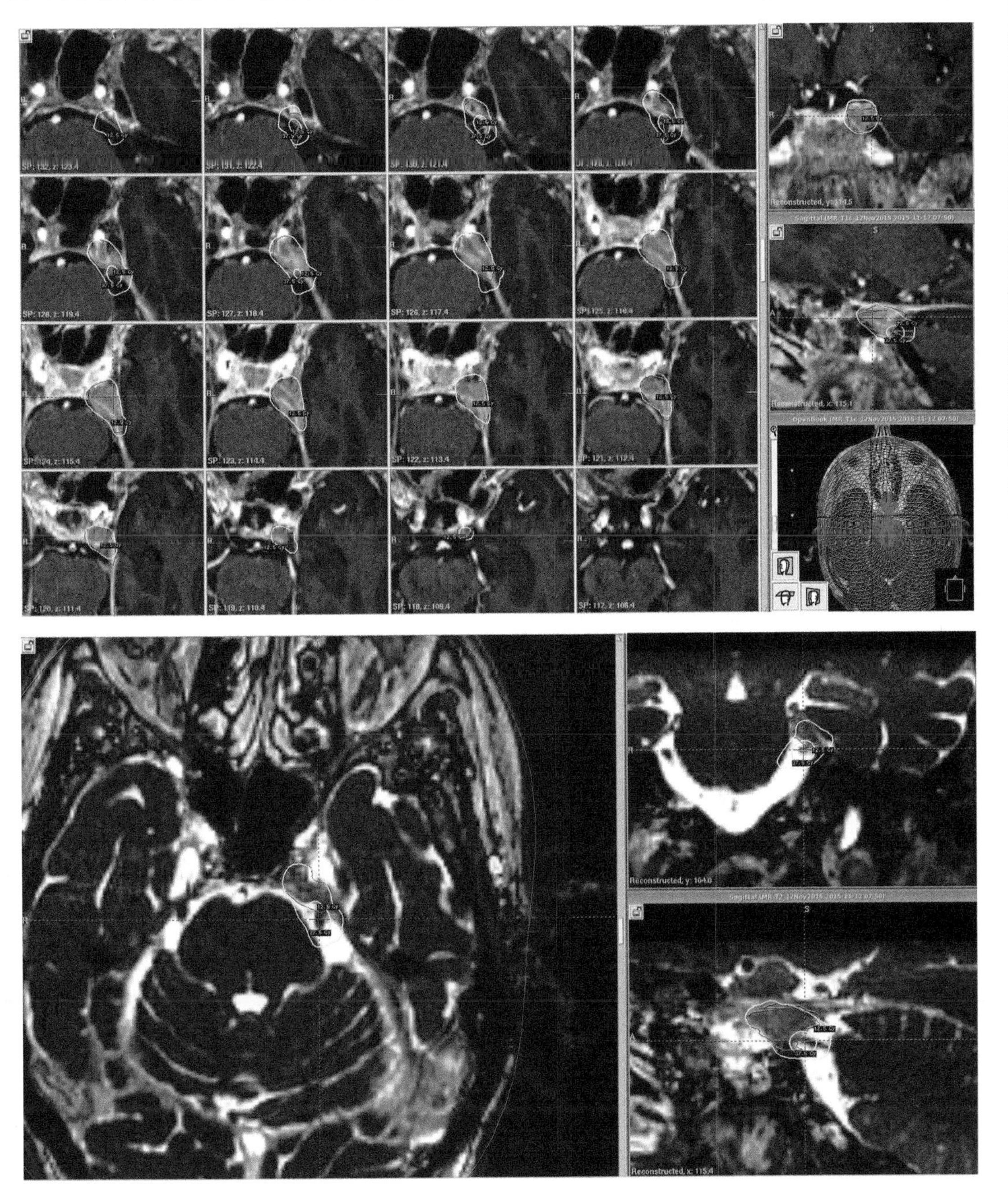

Fig. 2. Treatment plan targeting both the left trigeminal nerve and a petrocavernous meningioma.

Inventory-55 before and after GKS, Regis and colleagues[24] reported improvements across several QOL dimensions, including health perception, energy/fatigue, social function, emotional well-being, cognitive function, physical function, pain, and overall QOL. In another study, most patients (87.7%) reported they would recommend GKS to another patient.[27] Little and colleagues[36] found that 73% of patients reported no effect of TN on daily activities after GKS, and 72% reported that their TN did not affect their enjoyment of life post-GKS. A TN-specific QOL tool was devised by Knafo and colleagues.[37] In their study looking at patient-rated functional status in everyday life, patients reported significant improvements in QOL (return to work, performing normal daily activities, social life, pain free) by 6 months after radiosurgery.[37]

TUMOR-ASSOCIATED TRIGEMINAL NEURALGIA: A NOVEL TREATMENT APPROACH

Benign tumors of the skull base (eg, meningiomas, schwannomas, epidermoid cysts) can encroach onto the trigeminal nerve causing facial pain symptoms similar to that experienced by patients with idiopathic TN. Tumor-related facial pain underlies approximately 1% to 15% of patients with symptoms of TN.[38–40] Tumor-associated TN tends to be recalcitrant to medical management, and surgical resection is often favored. However, older patients or patients with multiple comorbidities may not be appropriate candidates for surgery. Achievement of pain relief following GKS that targets the tumor, conventionally at a median dose of 12 Gy, occurs in approximately 25% to 96% of patients, a much more modest effect than with idiopathic TN.[41–46] Tumor volume reduction was associated with decreased facial pain in one study,[45] however, not in another study.[46]

A novel treatment approach for tumor-related facial pain consists of targeting the nerve with a high-dose isocenter at a maximum of 75 to 80 Gy, followed by placement of down-weighted isocenters to summate the radiation dose over the remainder of the tumor to a mean margin dose of 12 Gy (**Figs. 1** and **2**). The long-term pain-relief outcomes of the combination of treating the nerve along with the tumor have yet to be determined.

SUMMARY

GKS is a safe and effective treatment approach for patients with TN and the least invasive surgical option. Longer-term data are now available from numerous international centers, demonstrating good pain-free rates in patients with type I TN, even past 5 years. Studies have also demonstrated that GKS remains effective even after a second, and potentially, a third GKS with minimal increase in complications.

The selection of patients to undergo GKS in the management of medically refractory TN has evolved over the last decade. Traditionally, patients that underwent GKS for TN were older patients with medical comorbidities and poor performance status, for whom more invasive procedures are contraindicated. However, an increasing number of patients are favoring GKS over more invasive approaches in order to avoid a general anesthetic, a prolonged hospital stay, and a higher risk of complications.

REFERENCES

1. Leksell L. Sterotaxic radiosurgery in trigeminal neuralgia. Acta Chir Scand 1971;137(4):311–4.
2. Kondziolka D, Lunsford LD, Flickinger JC, et al. Stereotactic radiosurgery for trigeminal neuralgia: a multiinstitutional study using the gamma unit. J Neurosurg 1996;84(6):940–5.
3. Rand RW, Jacques DB, Melbye RW, et al. Leksell Gamma Knife treatment of tic douloureux. Stereotact Funct Neurosurg 1993;61(Suppl 1):93–102.
4. Régis J, Manera L, Dufour H, et al. Effect of the Gamma Knife on trigeminal neuralgia. Stereotact Funct Neurosurg 1995;64(Suppl 1):182–92.
5. Regis J, Tuleasaca C, Resseguier N, et al. Long-term safety and efficacy of Gamma Knife surgery in classical trigeminal neuralgia: a 497-patient historical cohort study. J Neurosurg 2015;1–9. http://dx.doi.org/10.3171/2015.2.JNS142144.
6. Lucas JT, Nida AM, Isom S, et al. Predictive nomogram for the durability of pain relief from gamma knife radiation surgery in the treatment of trigeminal neuralgia. Int J Radiat Oncol Biol Phys 2014;89(1):120–6.
7. Marshall K, Chan MD, McCoy TP, et al. Predictive variables for the successful treatment of trigeminal neuralgia with gamma knife radiosurgery. Neurosurgery 2012;70(3):566–72.
8. Kondziolka D, Zorro O, Lobato-Polo J, et al. Gamma Knife stereotactic radiosurgery for idiopathic trigeminal neuralgia. J Neurosurg 2010;112(4):758–65.
9. Barker FG, Jannetta PJ, Bissonette DJ, et al. The long-term outcome of microvascular decompression for trigeminal neuralgia. N Engl J Med 1996;334(17):1077–83.
10. Sindou M, Leston J, Decullier E, et al. Microvascular decompression for primary trigeminal neuralgia: long-term effectiveness and prognostic factors in a

series of 362 consecutive patients with clear-cut neurovascular conflicts who underwent pure decompression. J Neurosurg 2007;107(6):1144–53.
11. Henson CF, Goldman HW, Rosenwasser RH, et al. Glycerol rhizotomy versus gamma knife radiosurgery for the treatment of trigeminal neuralgia: an analysis of patients treated at one institution. Int J Radiat Oncol Biol Phys 2005;63(1):82–90.
12. Brisman R. Microvascular decompression vs. gamma knife radiosurgery for typical trigeminal neuralgia: preliminary findings. Stereotact Funct Neurosurg 2007;85(2–3):94–8.
13. Pollock BE, Schoeberl KA. Prospective comparison of posterior fossa exploration and stereotactic radiosurgery dorsal root entry zone target as primary surgery for patients with idiopathic trigeminal neuralgia. Neurosurgery 2010;67(3):633–8 [discussion: 638–9].
14. Maesawa S, Salame C, Flickinger JC, et al. Clinical outcomes after stereotactic radiosurgery for idiopathic trigeminal neuralgia. J Neurosurg 2001; 94(1):14–20.
15. Young RF, Vermeulen SS, Grimm P, et al. Gamma Knife radiosurgery for treatment of trigeminal neuralgia: idiopathic and tumor related. Neurology 1997; 48(3):608–14.
16. Pollock BE, Phuong LK, Gorman DA, et al. Stereotactic radiosurgery for idiopathic trigeminal neuralgia. J Neurosurg 2002;97(2):347–53.
17. Mousavi SH, Niranjan A, Huang MJ, et al. Early radiosurgery provides superior pain relief for trigeminal neuralgia patients. Neurology 2015;85:1–8.
18. Rogers CL, Shetter AG, Ponce FA, et al. Gamma knife radiosurgery for trigeminal neuralgia associated with multiple sclerosis. J Neurosurg 2002; 97(Suppl 5):529–32.
19. Weller M, Marshall K, Lovato JF, et al. Single-institution retrospective series of gamma knife radiosurgery in the treatment of multiple sclerosis-related trigeminal neuralgia: factors that predict efficacy. Stereotact Funct Neurosurg 2014;92(1):53–8.
20. Zorro O, Lobato-Polo J, Kano H, et al. Gamma knife radiosurgery for multiple sclerosis-related trigeminal neuralgia. Neurology 2009;73(14):1149–54.
21. Brisman R, Khandji AG, Mooij RB. Trigeminal nerve-blood vessel relationship as revealed by high-resolution magnetic resonance imaging and its effect on pain relief after gamma knife radiosurgery for trigeminal neuralgia. Neurosurgery 2002;50(6): 1261–6 [discussion: 1266–7].
22. Ko AL, Lee A, Raslan AM, et al. Trigeminal neuralgia without neurovascular compression presents earlier than trigeminal neuralgia with neurovascular compression. J Neurosurg 2015;123(6):1519–27.
23. Matsuda S, Nagano O, Serizawa T, et al. Trigeminal nerve dysfunction after Gamma Knife surgery for trigeminal neuralgia: a detailed analysis. J Neurosurg 2010;113(Suppl):184–90.
24. Régis J, Metellus P, Hayashi M, et al. Prospective controlled trial of gamma knife surgery for essential trigeminal neuralgia. J Neurosurg 2006;104(6): 913–24.
25. Pollock BE, Phuong LK, Foote RL, et al. High-dose trigeminal neuralgia radiosurgery associated with increased risk of trigeminal nerve dysfunction. Neurosurgery 2001;49(1):58–62 [discussion 62–4].
26. Massager N, Lorenzoni J, Devriendt D, et al. Gamma knife surgery for idiopathic trigeminal neuralgia performed using a far-anterior cisternal target and a high dose of radiation. J Neurosurg 2004; 100(4):597–605.
27. Young B, Shivazad A, Kryscio RJ, et al. Long-term outcome of high-dose Gamma Knife surgery in treatment of trigeminal neuralgia. J Neurosurg 2013; 119(5):1166–75.
28. Massager N, Murata N, Tamura M, et al. Influence of nerve radiation dose in the incidence of trigeminal dysfunction after trigeminal neuralgia radiosurgery. Neurosurgery 2007;60(4):681–7 [discussion: 687–8].
29. Flickinger JC, Pollock BE, Kondziolka D, et al. Does increased nerve length within the treatment volume improve trigeminal neuralgia radiosurgery? A prospective double-blind, randomized study. Int J Radiat Oncol Biol Phys 2001;51(2):449–54.
30. Villavicencio AT, Lim M, Burneikiene S, et al. Cyberknife radiosurgery for trigeminal neuralgia treatment: a preliminary multicenter experience. Neurosurgery 2008;62(3):647–55 [discussion: 647–55].
31. Tuleasca C, Carron R, Resseguier N, et al. Repeat Gamma Knife surgery for recurrent trigeminal neuralgia: long-term outcomes and systematic review. J Neurosurg 2014;121(Suppl):210–21.
32. Park KJ, Kondziolka D, Berkowitz O, et al. Repeat gamma knife radiosurgery for trigeminal neuralgia. Neurosurgery 2012;70(2):295–305 [discussion: 305].
33. Helis CA, Lucas JT, Bourland JD, et al. Repeat radiosurgery for trigeminal neuralgia. Neurosurgery 2015; 77(5):755–61.
34. Tempel ZJ, Chivukula S, Monaco EA, et al. The results of a third Gamma Knife procedure for recurrent trigeminal neuralgia. J Neurosurg 2015;122(1):169–79.
35. Longhi M, Rizzo P, Nicolato A, et al. Gamma knife radiosurgery for trigeminal neuralgia: results and potentially predictive parameters–part I: idiopathic trigeminal neuralgia. Neurosurgery 2007;61(6): 1254–60 [discussion: 1260–1].
36. Little AS, Shetter AG, Shetter ME, et al. Long-term pain response and quality of life in patients with typical trigeminal neuralgia treated with gamma knife stereotactic radiosurgery. Neurosurgery 2008; 63(5):915–23 [discussion: 923–4].
37. Knafo H, Kenny B, Mathieu D. Trigeminal neuralgia: outcomes after gamma knife radiosurgery. Can J Neurol Sci 2009;36(1):78–82.

38. Bullitt E, Tew JM, Boyd J. Intracranial tumors in patients with facial pain. J Neurosurg 1986;64(6):865–71.
39. Nomura T, Ikezaki K, Matsushima T, et al. Trigeminal neuralgia: differentiation between intracranial mass lesions and ordinary vascular compression as causative lesions. Neurosurg Rev 1994;17(1):51–7.
40. Cheng TM, Cascino TL, Onofrio BM. Comprehensive study of diagnosis and treatment of trigeminal neuralgia secondary to tumors. Neurology 1993;43(11):2298–302.
41. Tanaka S, Pollock BE, Stafford SL, et al. Stereotactic radiosurgery for trigeminal pain secondary to benign skull base tumors. World Neurosurg 2013;80(3–4):371–7.
42. Squire SE, Chan MD, Furr RM, et al. Gamma knife radiosurgery in the treatment of tumor-related facial pain. Stereotact Funct Neurosurg 2012;90(3):145–50.
43. Régis J, Metellus P, Dufour H, et al. Long-term outcome after gamma knife surgery for secondary trigeminal neuralgia. J Neurosurg 2001;95(2):199–205.
44. Pollock BE, Iuliano BA, Foote RL, et al. Stereotactic radiosurgery for tumor-related trigeminal pain. Neurosurgery 2000;46(3):576–82 [discussion: 582–3].
45. Huang CF, Tu HT, Liu WS, et al. Gamma Knife surgery for trigeminal pain caused by benign brain tumors. J Neurosurg 2008;109(Suppl):154–9.
46. Kano H, Awan NR, Flannery TJ, et al. Stereotactic radiosurgery for patients with trigeminal neuralgia associated with petroclival meningiomas. Stereotact Funct Neurosurg 2011;89(1):17–24.

Endoscopic and Microscopic Microvascular Decompression

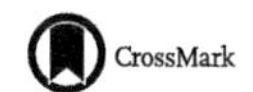

Matthew Piazza, MD[a], John Y.K. Lee, MD, MSCE[b,*]

KEYWORDS

- Endoscopic microvascular decompression • Trigeminal neuralgia • Neuroendoscopy
- Skull-base surgery • Microvascular decompression

KEY POINTS

- The endoscope provides enhanced visualization and illumination of lateral skull-base structures. The endoscope can be used to view neurovascular structures not seen by the microscope in microvascular decompression (MVD) surgery.
- The endoscope can be used as an adjunct to the microscope in MVD surgery, for example, endoscope-assisted MVD.
- Fully endoscopic MVD using an endoscope holder allows the surgeon to operate with 2 hands while retaining the panoramic views afforded by the endoscope.
- Adopting the "triangle" method to orient and introduce instruments, with the endoscope positioned at the apex, allows for safe passage of instrumentation into the operative field and avoidance of instrument clash.
- Meticulous hemostasis throughout the case is necessary because bleeding can obscure the view of the endoscope.

INTRODUCTION

Microvascular decompression (MVD) is a well-established and effective treatment of trigeminal neuralgia, hemifacial spasm, glossopharyngeal neuralgia, and other associated surgically treated craniofacial pain syndromes.[1,2] Traditionally, this surgery is performed under microscopic guidance through a retrosigmoid craniotomy. Treatment failures do occur and can be associated with inadequate visualization of the surgical anatomy—in particular, the point of contact of the offending vessel to the root entry zone.[3] This observation reflects an underlying problem with visualization provided by the microscope. Namely, the visualization of the anatomy of interest requires a direct line of sight with the light source when using the microscope. The incorporation of the endoscope into the armamentarium of the neurosurgeon has revolutionized anterior and ventral skull-base neurosurgery. The endoscope was first introduced as an alternative to the microscope in transsphenoidal pituitary surgery.[4] Its use was quickly expanded to approach lesions of the anterior skull base, tuberculum sella, and the clivus.[5–8] More recently, endoscopic approaches have been developed for use in lateral skull-base surgery, and in particular, in the surgical treatment of trigeminal neuralgia.[9–11] In this article, the fully endoscopic microvascular decompression (E-MVD) for patients with trigeminal neuralgia is discussed.

Disclosure Statement: The authors have nothing to disclose.
[a] Department of Neurosurgery, Hospital of the University of Pennsylvania, Perelman School of Medicine at the University of Pennsylvania, 3400 Spruce Street, 3rd Floor Silverstein, Philadelphia, PA 19104, USA; [b] Department of Neurosurgery, Pennsylvania Hospital, Perelman School of Medicine at the University of Pennsylvania, 235 South 8th Street, Washington Square West Building, Philadelphia, PA 19106, USA
* Corresponding author.
E-mail address: john.lee3@uphs.upenn.edu

Neurosurg Clin N Am 27 (2016) 305–313
http://dx.doi.org/10.1016/j.nec.2016.02.008

neurosurgery.theclinics.com

TECHNICAL AND ANATOMIC CONSIDERATIONS OF CEREBELLOPONTINE ANGLE ENDOSCOPIC SURGERY

There are several principal advantages of the endoscope over the microscope in cerebellopontine angle (CPA) base surgery. First, the endoscope allows for a panoramic and uninhibited view of surrounding anatomy. Unlike the microscope, which requires a direct line of site from the lens to the point of interest for optimal visualization, the endoscope has a field of view of approximately 90° from the tip of the endoscope (45° on each side from the axis of entry). This field of view allows the surgeon to see beyond the typical field of view of the dural opening, which in the case of the endoscopic MVD is quite small. This enhanced visualization can allow a complete understanding of the course of vessels and nerves from the point of origin to where they terminate or exit through the skull base. Second, the endoscope provides unparalleled illumination of the operative field. Finally, smaller exposures and less brain retraction are possible with the endoscope because of these latter 2 qualities, reducing potential morbidity for the patient.

Several investigators have attempted to rigorously evaluate the visualization benefits of the endoscope over the microscope for the retrosigmoid approach. Tang and colleagues[12] quantitatively assessed the visual field of the microscope versus the endoscope in a cadaver and found that the 30° endoscope offered a significantly larger field of view (nearly 2-fold) compared with the microscope. In another cadaveric study, Tang and colleagues[13] developed a numerical grading score for assessing maneuverability and demonstrated that endoscopic-assisted microsurgical MVD had superior scores compared with the microscope both with and without sacrificing the superior petrosal vein. Moreover, the endoscopy scores did not improve with taking the vein, in contrast to microscopy, suggesting an endoscopic approach may decrease the need to compromise the superior petrosal vein. In a detailed anatomic study, Takemura and colleagues[14] demonstrated that the endoscope had superior visualization of the skull-base meati and root entry zones into the brainstem of the cranial nerves and their relationship to surrounding vessels when compared with the microscope.

There is also ample evidence within the clinical literature regarding the benefits afforded by endoscopic visualization. Jarrahy and colleagues[15] performed MVD on 21 patients initially with the microscope; the endoscope was used to confirm the presence of offending vessels initially identified with the microscope and assess the adequacy of the decompression. Interestingly, 14 of the 51 offending vessels were only identified after the endoscope was introduced, and in 5 patients, further decompression was needed after it was deemed inadequate using the endoscope. In another study of patients undergoing MVD initially with the microscope alone, the endoscope was able to better delineate arterial anatomy in 25% of patients and detect vessels completely missed with microscopy in 8% of patients.[16] Rak and colleagues[17] found that the adjunctive use of the endoscope resulted in visualization and subsequent sacrifice of the trigeminal vein compressing the trigeminal nerve at the entrance of Meckel's cave in several patients within their series; in these cases, bone obscured the full view of the trigeminal nerve from the microscope. In their large case series of endoscopic assisted MVD (EA-MVD), Chen and colleagues[18] discovered vessel-nerve conflicts in 14.7% of their 167 patients only after using the endoscope. Indeed, the senior surgeon (J.Y.K.L.) has found the endoscope invaluable at detecting nerve-vessel contacts that would not otherwise be directly within the line of site of traditional means of visualization (**Figs. 1** and **2**).

Despite these advantages, the endoscope has not been widely adopted for lateral skull-base surgery for several reasons. The anatomy of the CPA requires delicate manipulation. Unlike endonasal approaches, where the structures encountered largely consist of mucosa, the sinuses, and bone, lateral skull-base surgery requires that the surgeon navigate neural tissues and blood vessels without causing injury; this is further complicated by the fact that the planes of access are largely potential spaces in contrast to the well-aerated spaces within the nasosinal cavities encountered in endonasal surgery. Although visualization of operative anatomy may be superior with the endoscope, some studies have suggested that maneuverability may be limited when compared with the microscope.[12] Furthermore, because the endoscope only captures images anterior to its tip and is frequently deep within the surgical field, the absence of visualization behind the field of view makes inserting or removing instruments from the operative field dangerous, and extreme care must be taken to avoid injuring vessels or neural tissue. Finally, completely endoscopic surgery lacks the depth perception afforded by the binocular vision of the microscope. However, the adept endoscopic surgeon can use

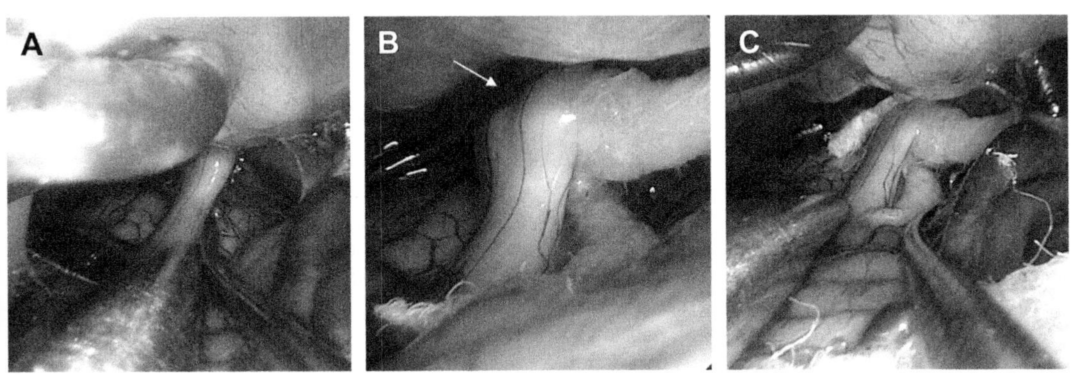

Fig. 1. Endoscope identifies additional point of compression from lateral vein along Meckel cave in a case of MVD for trigeminal neuralgia. (*A*) Typical view of dissection of the superior cerebellar artery (SCA) off of the trigeminal nerve. (*B*) Once the Teflon pad is placed between the SCA and the trigeminal nerve, the scope was advanced to reveal a compressive vein (*arrow*) lateral along Meckel cave. (*C*) View of trigeminal complex after decompression complete. Note that the endoscope afforded a complete view of the trigeminal nerve and allowed identification multiple points of vessel nerve contact.

visual cues from gentle manipulation of surrounding structures to create 3-dimensional representation of the anatomy. Furthermore, advances in stereoscopic high-definition optics are improving, and once optimized for use in CPA surgery, will likely become widely adopted and enhance surgeon dexterity. Nevertheless, in skilled hands, CPA surgery can be facilitated

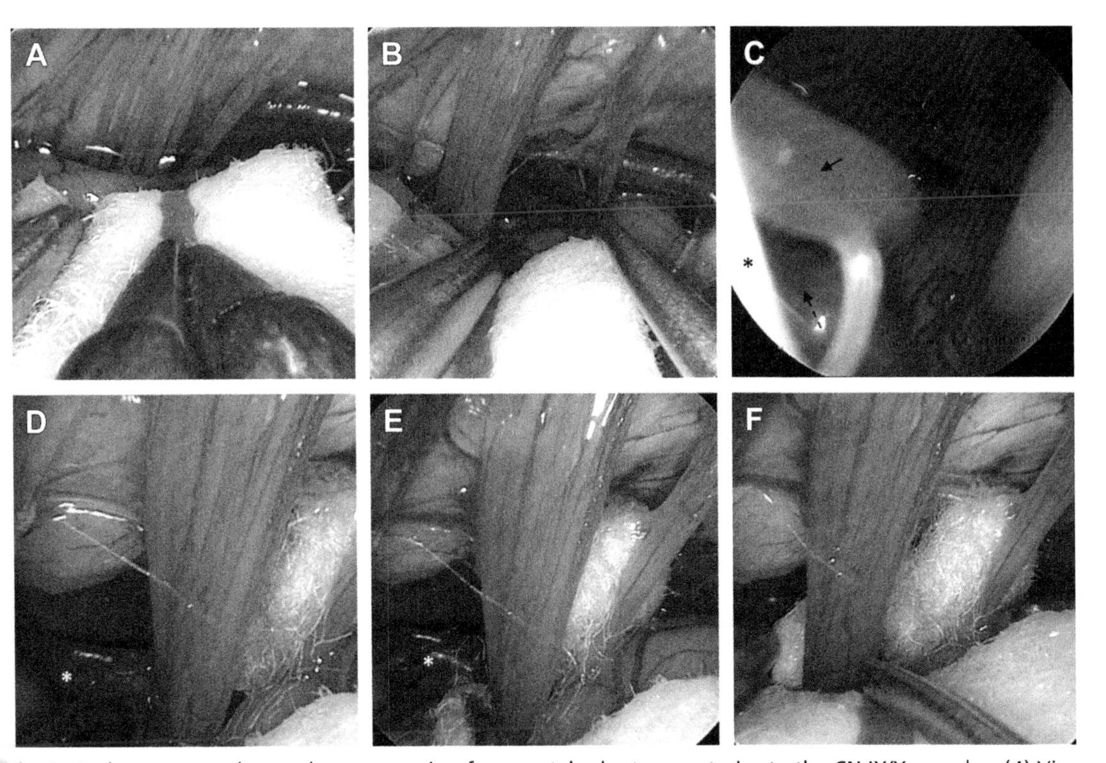

Fig. 2. Endoscope reveals vascular compression from vertebral artery posterior to the CN IX/X complex. (*A*) View of CN IX/X complex and offending anterior inferior cerebellar artery (AICA) after arachnoid dissection. (*B, C*) Dissection of AICA opens a window through which the endoscope is advanced, revealing vascular compression from vertebral artery (*dotted arrow*) and potentially posterior inferior cerebellar artery (PICA; *solid arrow*) of the nerve complex (*asterisk*). (*D*) Further dissection on the contralateral side of the nerve further delineates the vertebral artery (*asterisk*) and develops a plane through which Teflon is advanced (*E*). (*F*) Final view after Teflon is positioned posterior to the nerve complex but anterior to the compressive vertebral artery and PICA.

using the endoscope either as an adjunct to the microscope or as the sole source of illumination and visualization.

PATIENT SELECTION AND PREOPERATIVE WORKUP

In general, the indications for E-MVD are similar to those for microscopic MVD. The most common clinically entity requiring MVD in the United States is trigeminal neuralgia, although similar approaches are used for glossopharyngeal neuralgia, geniculate neuralgia, hemi-facial spasm, and vestibular nerve sectioning. Although the diagnosis and initial management of trigeminal neuralgia and associated peripheral neuropathies are discussed elsewhere in this text, they are briefly reviewed in **Table 1**.

Once the diagnosis of trigeminal neuralgia is made clinically, the patient should undergo imaging with MRI to rule out structural causes of trigeminal pain, although the low negative predictive value obviates the clinical utility of imaging for operative decision-making.[19] Interestingly, imaging may prove useful for the surgeon in deciding whether to use the endoscope. Sandell and colleagues[20] examined the utility of preoperative MRI in predicting the need for endoscopic assistance during a microscopic MVD to visualize the offending vessel. The investigators found an association with the fraction of microscopically visible nerve on preoperative MRI and the need for the endoscope, quoting an optimal cutoff of less than 35% of visible nerve. In addition to imaging, patients should undergo the typical preoperative laboratory assessment and, as this is an elective procedure, should be medically cleared for surgery. Before undergoing surgery, the patient's level of pain should be graded in a rigorous manner using a pain scale, such as the Brief Pain Inventory–Facial, to accurately assess outcomes postoperatively.[21,22]

OPERATIVE TECHNIQUE

Patient positioning and opening have been well described in the literature and is reviewed briefly here. The patient is taken to the operating room and placed under general anesthesia. The patient is placed in the Mayfield head clamp and positioned laterally with an axillary roll. The head is gently flexed and slightly rotated to the contralateral side; the position of the vertex relative to the floor is dictated by the cranial nerves of interest. It is kept parallel to the floor when performing MVD of the trigeminal nerve and dropped approximately 15° for decompression of the lower cranial nerves.[23] The following anatomic landmarks are useful to identify for planning burr hole and incision: the course of the transverse and sigmoid sinuses, the insertion of the digastric muscle, and the tip of the mastoid process. A line is typically drawn from the inion to the external auditory meatus to approximate the course of the transverse sinus; a similar line is drawn along the posterior aspect of the mastoid process for the sigmoid sinus (**Fig. 3**A). The burr hole is typically centered just inferior and posterior to the intersection of these 2 lines, and the incision is planned accordingly. Before preparation and draping, the surgeon should position the pneumatic holding arm for the endoscope. The pneumatic arm is attached to the most cephalad aspect of the patient bed, which usually requires placing the arm board just inferior to this attachment. The pneumatic arm is arranged in a figure 4, with the distal joint of the arm positioned directly above the planned craniectomy site.

Once the patient is prepared and draped, an approximately 4-cm linear skin incision is made

Table 1
Craniofacial pain syndromes

Syndrome	Involved Cranial Nerve	Most Common Offending Vessel	Distribution of Pain
Trigeminal neuralgia	CNV	SCA	Forehead, upper eyelid, scalp (V1); lower eyelid, cheek, upper lip (V2); jaw, lower lip (V3)
Geniculate neuralgia	CN VII	AICA	Deep ear, eye/orbit, cheek, nasal/palatal pain; occasional salivation, taste disturbances, tinnitus, vertiginous symptoms; may be accompanied by hemifacial spasm
Glossopharyngeal neuralgia	CN IX/X	PICA	Throat and base of tongue, radiating to ear and neck; salivating/coughing possible; autonomic symptoms rare

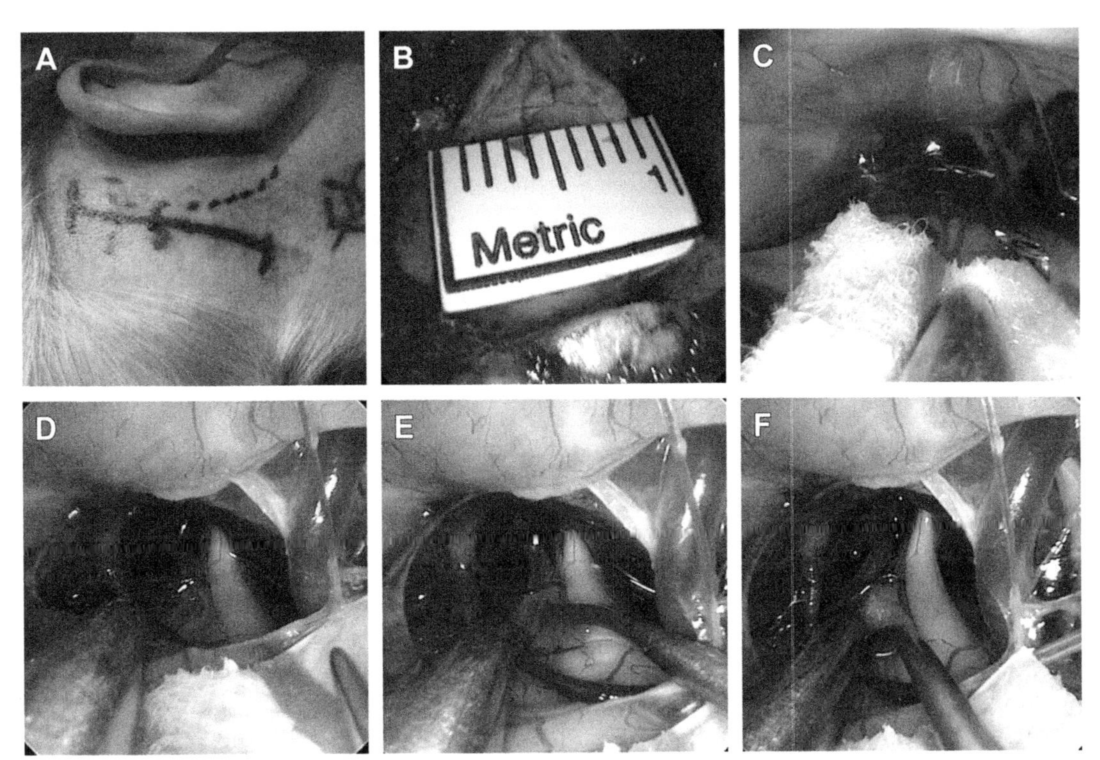

Fig. 3. Key technical steps in fully E-MVD. (*A*) Planned incision with for retrosigmoid craniotomy for MVD. Note the dotted lines represent the approximate location of the transverse and sigmoid sinuses. (*B*) Once retrosigmoid craniectomy is performed, an approximately 1-cm C-shaped dural incision is made and reflected anteriorly. (*C*) The cerebellum is gently retracted, and sharp dissection is used to open the arachnoid to allow CSF egress to facilitate brain relaxation. (*D*) Once brain relaxation is achieved, the trigeminal nerve complex is visualized and the offending SCA is identified. (*E*) A microdissector is used to develop a plane between the SCA and the trigeminal nerve. (*F*) Once an adequate plane is developed between the vessel and the nerve, a Teflon pad is introduced to complete the MVD. Note the "triangle" method used here, with the endoscope at the apex, instruments arranged parallel to the endoscope, and the cottonoid for safe introduction into the operative field and avoidance of instrument clashing.

just inferior to the junction of the transverse and sigmoid sinuses and approximately 1 cm behind the patient's hairline. This incision can be extended as needed. The fascia and muscle are dissected to bone, and a burr hole is made with a drill just above and medial to the most cephalad aspect of the digastric groove. The burr hole should be extended superiorly and anteriorly until the posterior and inferior borders of the sigmoid and transverse sinuses are visualized, respectively. Hemostasis is achieved, and any air cells encountered during bony exposure should be occluded with wax to prevent potential cerebrospinal fluid (CSF) leak. Next, an approximately 1-cm-wide C-shaped dural opening is made and reflected anteriorly (**Fig. 3**B). The pneumatic holding arm and endoscope are brought into position. For the MVD, the authors prefer using the 2.7-mm 0° endoscope (Karl Storz; El Segundo, CA, USA) because the smaller diameter facilitates the passage and manipulation of instruments through the dural opening. The smaller diameter scope also minimizes instrument clash. The image provided by the 2.7-mm endoscope is inferior to that of the typical 4-mm endoscope used frequently in endonasal skull-base surgery; however, with high-definition cameras, this limit is negligible. Angled endoscopes can be introduced later in the operation to facilitate visualization of the anatomy. To maximize safety and maneuverability, the endoscope should be positioned at the apex of an invisible, equilateral triangle, with the suction and microinstruments forming the lower left and right vertices, respectively.

Next, using a rectangular piece of Duraprene glove combined with a cottonoid patty to protect the cerebellum, the endoscope is inserted into the dural opening with gentle retraction on the cerebellum. Typically, the suction is placed in the nondominant hand to optimize dexterity with the microinstruments during dissection using the dominant hand. Sharp dissection is used to open the arachnoid of the medial CPA cistern and the cerebellomedullary cistern to allow CSF egress (**Fig. 3**C). This critical step should allow adequate brain relaxation to visualize the cranial nerves and creates a clear operative corridor (**Fig. 3**D). It is important in elderly patients to avoid rapid overdrainage because this can lead to sag and excessive stretch on vascular structures.

At this stage, the cranial nerves of interest are inspected and an offending vessel is usually identified. A microdissector is used to dissect and mobilize the vessel off of the cranial nerve. Throughout the microdissection portion of the case, it is crucial that instruments are passed through the dural opening in a consistent fashion (ie, the "triangle" approach) and parallel to the endoscope. To reiterate, the endoscope should always be oriented at the apex of the triangle, lying adjacent to the petrous bone and sigmoid sinus. There is both a distal and a proximal triangle to account for because the endoscope can sometimes be placed so that a perfect view of the anatomy is seen on the screen, but the endoscope crosses the working space at the level of the dural opening. By maintaining a strict equilateral triangle at both the proximal and the distal triangle, instrument clash is avoided. The cottonoid is a useful guide when inserting instrumentation into the field, especially when the endoscope is parked distally near the cranial nerve of interest. Maintaining the instruments at the base of the triangle is a natural position from a surgical perspective because the root entry zone typically resides in this location. In general, the authors prefer using instruments with gently curved tips because more aggressively curved instruments can prove dangerous when working near delicate vessels or nerves. In addition, the authors prefer the use of single-shaft instruments rather than conventional microinstruments. Conventionally, bayoneted instruments are generally too wide for the 1-cm dural opening into the CPA. Gentle retraction of the cerebellum can be employed using the suction held in the surgeon's nondominant hand while dissection is carried out. If the anatomy is difficult to visualize, using an angled endoscope is oftentimes useful because it may allow detection of a compressive vessel located outside the field of view of the 0° endoscope. The authors have found it particularly helpful for anatomic visualization in cases of hemifacial spasm or geniculate neuralgia. Once adequate mobilization of the offending vessel has been achieved, the vessel is dissected away from the nerve (**Fig. 3**E), and a Teflon pad is then placed in between it and the nerve of interest (**Fig. 3**F), completing the MVD. If no clear offending vessel can be identified, a neurolysis or glycerol rhizotomy[24] is performed.

Throughout the procedure, meticulous hemostasis is imperative because bleeding can obscure visualization and can be difficult to control if not quickly addressed. Hence, careful microdissection and bipolar electrocautery are used throughout the case. Although this method avoids sacrificing major venous structures like the petrosal vein, there is a rare risk of venous stasis and cerebellar swelling. If the vein must be taken, the authors have found that moving the endoscope back allows for introduction of larger conventional instruments, like a bayoneted bipolar. Once hemostasis is achieved, the dura is closed. It is imperative that the closure be watertight and should be supplemented by muscle if needed. the authors sequentially place a piece of Duragen, dry Gelfoam, and a large burr hole cover over the craniectomy site to optimize the dural seal and prevent a CSF leak from forming. The wound is copiously irrigated and closed in a layered fashion.

ENDOSCOPIC-ASSISTED MICROVASCULAR DECOMPRESSION

Although completely endoscopic CPA surgery has a steep learning curve, one of the chief advantages of this approach is that 2-handed surgery is possible while having optimal visualization. However, for those surgeons who are more facile using the microscope, the endoscope can still serve as a tool for understanding the anatomy. In these cases, bimanual surgery is performed under the microscope until after dissection of the arachnoid. At this point, when greater visualization of neurovascular structures needed, the endoscope can be used. Because the usual focusing distance of the microscope is 375 mm, it has to be moved either completely out of the field or the focal length has to be increased in order for the endoscope to be brought into the field. If the endoscope is to be used primarily for enhanced visualization, then it can be introduced using 2 hands, and the surgeon can revert to the microscope and rely on memory once he or she has adequately surveyed and understood the anatomy. If the surgeon wishes to operate using the endoscope at this stage, he or she can adopt a one-handed technique with the endoscope and use microinstruments or suction in the other hand; there are, however, significant restrictions to maneuverability with this approach. Some surgeons have attached a microsuction device to the endoscope to facilitate one-handed surgery, although there are inherent issues with image motion with any attempt to locally suction.[25] Despite these limitations, endoscopy remains a useful adjunct for surgeons who heavily rely on the microscope within their practice.

MICROSCOPIC MICROVASCULAR DECOMPRESSION

Dr Jannetta's introduction of the microscope to the surgical procedure allowed for excellent illumination and magnification beginning with his first case report in 1967.[26] Since that time and over the past fifty years, the microscopic microvascular decompression has become routine, safe, and effective surgery.[27,28] The procedure is much the same as described in the preceding paragraphs except that that the dural opening is usually slightly larger in order to provide more exposure and light entrance into the cerebellopontine angle.

There are some advantages of the microscope as compared to the endoscope. Specifically, the microscope allows three dimensional visualization, albeit at the expense of depth of field as only a narrow sliver of depth is in focus at the magnifications generally needed for successful MVD. In addition, the microscope is commonly used by generations of neurosurgeons and thus comfort is high. Another advantage is that the microscope does not experience condensation on the optical apparatus as it is not immersed in the body cavity.

There are disadvantages of the microscope, however. Because of the difficulty in seeing nuances of anatomy, Dr Jannetta had suggested use of an angled dental mirror in order to see around corners.[29] This is obviously not necessary when performing fully endoscopic or endoscope-assisted microvascular decompression. The use of a retractor is user dependent and has not necessarily been proven to result in more ischemia to the cerebellum, but in general most microscopic MVDs are performed with adjunct use of cerebellar retractors. As evidenced by fifty years of publications, the microscopic MVD is a standard and routine procedure advocated by many experienced neurosurgeons, and we continue to recommend its use for individuals not familiar with endoscopic techniques.

POTENTIAL PITFALLS AND BAILOUT

The most common risks associated with endoscopic MVD are related to the surgeon's familiarity with the endoscope. If technical difficulties are encountered with the endoscope, the surgeon should convert to the usual microscopic MVD. If the anatomy is difficult to visualize using the 0° endoscope, the angled endoscopes may be used to provide an additional view. However, a common pitfall among those surgeons not familiar with the endoscope is that what is visualized cannot always be safely reached with instruments, and the surgeon should be mindful of this limitation when using the endoscope. Bleeding, if not controlled in a timely fashion, can obscure the view from the endoscope tip; intermittent irrigation of the lens tip can clear the field of view, but timely control with bleeding using bipolar electrocautery and hemostatic agents is paramount.

POSTOPERATIVE CARE AND COMPLICATIONS

Postoperative care for endoscopic MVDs is similar to that after the microscopic MVD. Patients spend a night in the neurosurgical intensive care unit for observation and are transferred to the neurosurgical floor on postoperative day 1. Imaging is not obtained unless patients have a neurologic change. Patients may complain of headache, neck stiffness or spasm, nausea, and vomiting and should be treated symptomatically. Patients usually are discharged on postoperative day 2 or 3.

COMPLICATIONS

Complications are similar to that of the microscopic MVD and include infection, CSF leak, pseudomeningocele formation, hemorrhage, cerebellar injury or stroke, cranial nerve injury (transient or permanent), and rarely, death. Careful attention to hemostasis intraoperatively can minimize the risk of postoperative hemorrhage. Aggressive retraction of the cerebellum can lead to cerebellar contusion, vascular injury, or stretch on the cranial nerves, and the authors advocate for using intermittent, gentle retraction of the cerebellum with the suction for fully endoscopic MVD. CN VIII is at greatest risk of injury, and implementing intraoperative neuromonitoring, specifically with brainstem auditory evoked potentials, may reduce the risk of hearing loss postoperatively. CSF leak can be avoided by occlusion of mastoid air cells with bone wax if encountered on opening and watertight dural closure. Occasionally, the dura cannot be repaired primarily; in these cases, the authors recommend, and have had good results, using a muscle patch followed by layered application of dural substitute and Gelfoam.

OUTCOMES

As of October 2015, the senior author (J.Y.K.L.) has performed 199 fully E-MVD, 83% of which were for trigeminal neuralgia, 17 EA-MVD, and 126 MVDs without an endoscope earlier in his experience. Although the outcomes are mostly short term, there have been no complications directly related to using the endoscope, and there have been no conversions to the microscope because of technical difficulties with the endoscope. The authors recently published their early experience with fully e-MVD for trigeminal neuralgia with promising results.[9] In this series of 47 consecutive patients undergoing E-MVD, there was again no morbidity attributable to using the endoscope, and patient outcomes were promising with 94% of patients endorsing improvement of preoperative symptoms. The authors are currently preparing a manuscript comparing results between E-MVD and conventional MVD, and identification of vessels is more successful with the use of the endoscope; however, early results demonstrate equivalent pain-free results. Interestingly, there appears to be less associated postoperative headache (manuscript pending).

Several other surgeons have published their experience with fully endoscopic MVDs. Kabil and colleagues[30] reported their large case series of 255 patients undergoing fully endoscopic MVDs and found that, in the subgroup of patients with long-term follow-up, 98% of patients had some relief (93% with complete relief). Their complication rate was also very low, with less than 1% of patients experiencing significant hearing loss, facial palsy, or severe facial numbness. They compared their incidence of complications with pooled incidences from several studies of microscopic MVD and found that endoscopic MVD had lower rates of complications in all categories. In their series of 51 patients who underwent E-MVD for trigeminal neuralgia, Yadav and colleagues[31] reported 94% of patients experiencing some relief of pain, with 90% of patients having complete relief. Their complication rate was relatively low, all of which were temporary, with only 2 patients having postoperative trigeminal dysesthesias and one patient each having facial paresis, decreased hearing, or vertiginous symptoms. Interestingly, the investigators compared their endoscopically treated patients with a historical EA-MVD cohort with overall lower frequency of complete pain relief (84%) and greater complication rates, including one patient with permanent facial paralysis and more frequent temporary cranial neuropathies. Setty and colleagues[32] published their series of E-MVD with similar results, reporting a 98% complete pain relief rate and no reported postoperative cranial neuropathies. Although larger, multicenter prospective studies are needed to compare outcomes and complications of endoscopic MVD with microscopic MVD, these data suggest that a purely endoscopic approach to MVD, in experienced hands, can result in excellent symptomatic relief with minimal complications.

SUMMARY

In conclusion, the endoscope offers unparalleled illumination and panoramic views of the CPA and can be either a useful adjunct or the sole source of visualization when surgically treating patients with trigeminal neuralgia or associated craniofacial pain syndromes. In skilled hands, use of the endoscope can lead to enhanced identification of offending vessels, minimal cerebellar retraction, and smaller craniotomy openings when compared with microscopic MVDs. Although larger, controlled prospective studies are needed to compare outcomes of endoscopic to microscopic MVDs, the authors expect widespread adoption of the endoscope into the skull-base neurosurgeon's armamentarium will allow him or her not only to surgically treat craniofacial pain syndromes effectively but also to tackle increasingly more complex skull-base abnormalities in a minimally invasive fashion.

REFERENCES

1. Jannetta PJ. Observations on the etiology of trigeminal neuralgia, hemifacial spasm, acoustic nerve dysfunction and glossopharyngeal neuralgia. Definitive microsurgical treatment and results in 117 patients. Neurochirurgia (Stuttg) 1977;20:145–54.
2. Barker FG, Jannetta PJ, Bissonette DJ, et al. The long-term outcome of microvascular decompression for trigeminal neuralgia. N Engl J Med 1996;334:1077–83.
3. Ugwuanyi UC, Kitchen ND. The operative findings in re-do microvascular decompression for recurrent trigeminal neuralgia. Br J Neurosurg 2010;24:26–30.
4. Jho HD, Carrau RL. Endoscopy assisted transsphenoidal surgery for pituitary adenoma. Technical note. Acta Neurochir (Wien) 1996;138:1416–25.
5. Lee JY, Ramakrishnan VR, Chiu AG, et al. Endoscopic endonasal surgical resection of tumors of the medial orbital apex and wall. Clin Neurol Neurosurg 2012;114:93–8.
6. Paluzzi A, Gardner P, Fernandez-Miranda JC, et al. The expanding role of endoscopic skull base surgery. Br J Neurosurg 2012;26:649–61.
7. Adappa ND, Learned KO, Palmer JN, et al. Radiographic enhancement of the nasoseptal flap does not predict postoperative cerebrospinal fluid leaks in endoscopic skull base reconstruction. Laryngoscope 2012;122:1226–34.
8. Adappa ND, Lee JYK, Chiu AG, et al. Olfactory groove meningioma. Otolaryngol Clin North Am 2011;44:965–80, ix.
9. Bohman L-E, Pierce J, Stephen JH, et al. Fully endoscopic microvascular decompression for trigeminal neuralgia: technique review and early outcomes. Neurosurg Focus 2014;37:E18.

10. Lang S-S, Chen HI, Lee JYK. Endoscopic microvascular decompression: a stepwise operative technique. ORL J Otorhinolaryngol Relat Spec 2012;74:293–8.
11. Halpern CH, Lang S-S, Lee JYK. Fully endoscopic microvascular decompression: our early experience. Minim Invasive Surg 2013;2013:739432.
12. Tang CT, Kurozumi K, Pillai P, et al. Quantitative analysis of surgical exposure and maneuverability associated with the endoscope and the microscope in the retrosigmoid and various posterior petrosectomy approaches to the petroclival region using computer tomograpy-based frameless stereotaxy. Clin Neurol Neurosurg 2013;115:1058–62.
13. Tang CT, Baidya NB, Ammirati M. Endoscope-assisted neurovascular decompression of the trigeminal nerve: a cadaveric study. Neurosurg Rev 2013;36:403–10.
14. Takemura Y, Inoue T, Morishita T, et al. Comparison of microscopic and endoscopic approaches to the cerebellopontine angle. World Neurosurg 2014;82:427–41.
15. Jarrahy R, Berci G, Shahinian HK. Endoscope-assisted microvascular decompression of the trigeminal nerve. Otolaryngol Head Neck Surg 2000;123:218–23.
16. Teo C, Nakaji P, Mobbs RJ. Endoscope-assisted microvascular decompression for trigeminal neuralgia: technical case report. Neurosurgery 2006;59:ONSE489–90 [discussion: ONSE490].
17. Rak R, Sekhar LN, Stimac D, et al. Endoscope-assisted microsurgery for microvascular compression syndromes. Neurosurgery 2004;54:876–81 [discussion: 881–3].
18. Chen MJ, Zhang WJ, Yang C, et al. Endoscopic neurovascular perspective in microvascular decompression of trigeminal neuralgia. J Craniomaxillofac Surg 2008;36:456–61.
19. Anderson VC, Berryhill PC, Sandquist MA, et al. High-resolution three-dimensional magnetic resonance angiography and three-dimensional spoiled gradient-recalled imaging in the evaluation of neurovascular compression in patients with trigeminal neuralgia: a double-blind pilot study. Neurosurgery 2006;58:666–73 [discussion: 666–73].
20. Sandell T, Ringstad GA, Eide PK. Usefulness of the endoscope in microvascular decompression for trigeminal neuralgia and MRI-based prediction of the need for endoscopy. Acta Neurochir (Wien) 2014;156:1901–9 [discussion: 1909].
21. Sandhu SK, Halpern CH, Vakhshori V, et al. Brief Pain Inventory–Facial minimum clinically important difference. J Neurosurg 2015;122:180–90.
22. Lee JYK, Chen HI, Urban C, et al. Development of and psychometric testing for the brief pain inventory-facial in patients with facial pain syndromes. J Neurosurg 2010;113:516–23.
23. McLaughlin MR, Jannetta PJ, Clyde BL, et al. Microvascular decompression of cranial nerves: lessons learned after 4400 operations. J Neurosurg 1999;90:1–8.
24. Goodwin CR, Yang JX, Bettegowda C, et al. Glycerol rhizotomy via a retrosigmoid approach as an alternative treatment for trigeminal neuralgia. Clin Neurol Neurosurg 2013;115:2454–6.
25. Cutler AR, Kaloostian SW, Ishiyama A, et al. Two-handed endoscopic-directed vestibular nerve sectioning: case series and review of the literature. J Neurosurg 2012;117:507–13.
26. Jannetta P. Arterial compression of the trigeminal nerve at the pons in patients with trigeminal neuralgia. J Neurosurg 1967;26(Suppl):159–62.
27. Sekula R, Frederickson A, Jannetta P, et al. Microvascular decompression for elderly patients with trigeminal neuralgia: a prospective study and systematic review with meta-analysis. J Neurosurg 2011;114:172–9.
28. Xia L, Zhong J, Zhu J, et al. Effectiveness and safety of microvascular decompression surgery for treatment of trigeminal neuralgia: a systematic review. J Craniofac Surg 2014;25:1413–7.
29. Jannetta P, McLaughlin M, Casey K. Technique of microvascular decompression: a technical note. Neurosurg Focus 2005;18:E5.
30. Kabil MS, Eby JB, Shahinian HK. Endoscopic vascular decompression versus microvascular decompression of the trigeminal nerve. Minim Invasive Neurosurg 2005;48:207–12.
31. Yadav YR, Parihar V, Agarwal M, et al. Endoscopic vascular decompression of the trigeminal nerve. Minim Invasive Neurosurg 2011;54:110–4.
32. Setty P, Volkov AA, D'Andrea KP, et al. Endoscopic vascular decompression for the treatment of trigeminal neuralgia: clinical outcomes and technical note. World Neurosurg 2014;81:603–8.

The Role of Imaging for Trigeminal Neuralgia

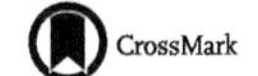

A Segmental Approach to High-Resolution MRI

Daniel P. Seeburg, MD, PhD, Benjamin Northcutt, MD, Nafi Aygun, MD, Ari M. Blitz, MD*

KEYWORDS

- Trigeminal neuralgia • Neurovascular contact • MRI

KEY POINTS

- High-resolution isotropic imaging allows detailed evaluation of nearly the entire course of the trigeminal nerve (cranial nerve [CN] V), from its brainstem nuclei to the distal branches of its 3 main divisions.
- Imaging in patients with trigeminal neuralgia (TGN) allows assessment for the presence, type, and degree of neurovascular contact in the cerebellopontine cistern.
- Imaging also allows evaluation for secondary causes of TGN, including multiple sclerosis (MS) as well as benign and malignant neoplasms.
- State-of-the-art MRI techniques, including diffusion tensor imaging (DTI) and functional MRI (fMRI), are providing insight into the pathogenesis of TGN.

INTRODUCTION

TGN is a rare unilateral episodic facial pain syndrome affecting the CN V and is characterized by paroxysmal lancinating shocklike pain attacks typically evoked by touch. With improvements in technology, the role of imaging in TGN has continued to evolve. High-resolution MRI now affords exquisite anatomic detail and allows radiologists to scrutinize nearly the entire course of CN V, from its nuclei in the brainstem to the distal branches of its 3 main divisions, the ophthalmic, maxillary, and mandibular nerves. This article focuses first on the normal MRI appearance of the course of CN V and how best to image each segment. Special attention is then devoted to the role of MRI in presurgical evaluation of patients with neurovascular conflict and in identifying the causes of TGN, including MS. Fundamental concepts in postsurgical imaging after neurovascular decompression are also addressed. Finally, how imaging has been used to better understand the etiology of TGN is discussed.

NORMAL MRI APPEARANCE OF THE TRIGEMINAL NERVE BY SEGMENT

CN V separates into 3 main divisions anteriorly as it exits the head: CN V.1—the ophthalmic division, CN V.2—the maxillary division, and CN V.3—the mandibular division. Each division subserves sensation to the face, with CN V.1, CN V.2, and CN V.3 responsible for sensation to the upper, middle, and lower thirds of the face, respectively.

Disclosure Statement: The authors have nothing to disclose.
Division of Neuroradiology, The Russel H. Morgan Department of Radiology and Radiologic Science, The Johns Hopkins Hospital, Phipps B-100, 600 North Wolfe Street, Baltimore, MD 21287, USA
* Corresponding author.
E-mail address: Ablitz1@jhmi.edu

Neurosurg Clin N Am 27 (2016) 315–326
http://dx.doi.org/10.1016/j.nec.2016.02.004

In addition, CN V.3 has a motor function, innervating the majority of the muscles of mastication. Imaging of CN V is now commonly performed using high-resolution isotropic 3-D MRI, replacing the standard 2-D techniques, and allowing for exquisite anatomic evaluation of CN V.

At the authors' institution, a dedicated protocol for assessment of TGN has been used for several years and in several hundred patients afflicted by TGN. The protocol includes isotropic sequences used for evaluation of the CNs, including precontrast and postcontrast constructive interference in the steady state (CISS) images, which use fast imaging in steady state free precession to render an image with mixed T1 and T2 weighting as well as precontrast and postcontrast volumetric interpolated breath-hold examination (VIBE), which is a type of T1-weighted gradient-recalled echo sequence. The authors' experience with CISS imaging, which affords the highest spatial resolution and the greatest anatomic detail, forms the basis for much of the following information.

Previous reviews by Blitz and colleagues[1,2] have defined a standardized nomenclature of the segments of the CNs, which is expanded for CN V in this article (**Box 1**, **Table 1**). The nuclei of the CN V (CN V.a) extend from the midbrain to the upper cervical spinal cord with the parenchymal fascicular segments (CN V.b) extending anteriorly toward the surface of the pons. A full review of the CN V.a and CN V.b segments is beyond the scope of this review, which focuses primarily on the components of CN V more readily accessible to the surgeon.

The apparent origin of the cisternal segment of CN V (CN V.c) is identified arising from the lateral aspect of the midpons (**Fig. 1**A). Anatomic studies have shown that there is a somatotopic organization to the trigeminal sensory root, with nerve fibers of the CN V.1 primarily rostral within the root, CN V.2 fibers comprising a greater medial portion of the root, and nerve fibers from the CN V.3 caudolateral within the root.[3] The apparent origin of the motor root(s) of CN V is/are often identified arising separately from the remainder of the CN V rootlets, located superior and medial to the apparent origin of the much larger sensory component of the nerve.[2]

CN V.c enters the dural cave of CN V (CN V.d) (Meckel's cave) through the porus trigeminus (see **Fig. 1**). Meckel's cave contains the gasserian (also known as the trigeminal or semilunar) ganglion, which is positioned along the anterior and inferior margin of Meckel's cave and can be identified on axial and sagittal precontrast CISS images (see **Fig. 1**A, B). The ganglion normally demonstrates enhancement on postcontrast imaging (see **Fig. 1**B, C). The remainder of CN V, however, should not show enhancement on postcontrast imaging. CN V divides distal to the gasserian ganglion into the CN V.1, CN V.2, and CN V.3 divisions (**Fig. 2**). (Note: the authors prefer the term, *CN V.1*, to reduce ambiguity with the abducens nerve, CN VI.)

The interdural segment of the V.1 nerve (V.1.e) extends along the lateral wall of the cavernous sinus superiorly and anteriorly toward the superior orbital fissure. The foraminal segment of the V.1 nerve (V.1.f) begins at the superior orbital fissure. It divides in the superior orbital fissure into the lacrimal and frontal branches superiorly and into the nasociliary branch inferiorly, which continue into the orbit as extraforaminal branches of CN V (V.1.g). The frontal nerve extends through supraorbital foramen, the lacrimal branch extends to the lacrimal gland, and nasociliary branches extend to the globe and nasal cavity.

The interdural segment of the V.2 nerve (V.2.e) travels below V.1.e along the lateral wall of the cavernous sinus (**Fig. 3**) and extends anteriorly as the foraminal segment (V.2.f) through the foramen rotundum. The extraforaminal segment (V.2.g) extends to the pterygopalatine ganglion, where it divides into the infraorbital nerve, which travels through the infraorbital foramen; the zygomatic nerve, which enters the orbit via the inferior orbital fissure and divides into the zygomaticofacial and zygomaticotemporal branches, the latter of which sends a small twig to the lacrimal nerve; and the

Box 1
Nomenclature of the anatomic segments of the cranial nerves used in this review, as detailed in the articles by Blitz and colleagues

a. Nuclear
b. Parenchymal fascicular
c. Cisternal
d. Dural cave
e. Interdural
f. Foraminal
g. Extraforaminal

Adapted from Blitz A, Choudhri A, Chonka Z, et al. Anatomic considerations, nomenclature, and advanced cross-sectional imaging techniques for visualization of the cranial nerve segments by MR imaging. Neuroimaging Clin N Am 2014;24(1):1–15; and Blitz A, Macedo L, Chonka Z, et al. High-resolution CISS MR imaging with and without contrast for evaluation of the upper cranial nerves. Neuroimaging Clin N Am 2014;24(1):17–34.

Table 1
Segmental delineation of the trigeminal nerve and key associated anatomic landmarks

Segment	Cisternal (V.c)	Dural Cave (V.d)	Interdural (V.e)	Foraminal (V.f)	Extraforaminal (V.g)
CN V	CN V root	Gasserian ganglion in Meckel's cave	—	—	—
CN V.1	—	—	Cavernous Sinus	Superior orbital fissure	Frontal, lacrimal, nasociliary nerves
CN V.2	—	—	Cavernous Sinus	Foramen rotundum	Pterygopalatine ganglion; infraorbital, zygomatic, superior alveolar nerves
CN V.3	—	—	Inconstantly seen	Foramen ovale	Motor branches to muscles of mastication; auriculotemporal, lingual, inferior alveolar nerves

Important branch nerves of the extraforaminal segments are listed in the final column.

superior alveolar nerves, which serve for sensation of the maxillary teeth.[4]

The V.3 interdural segment (V.3.e) is short and inconsistently seen as it passes inferiorly from Meckel's cave where it becomes the foraminal segment (V.3.f) within the foramen ovale. As with V.2.f, this is surrounded by extensive perineural vascular plexus, which allows the nerve to best be visualized on postcontrast images, such as postcontrast CISS (see **Figs. 2** and **3**). The extraforaminal segment (V.3.g) has several branches, of which the inferior alveolar nerve can commonly be seen extending to the mandibular foramen and motor branches to the muscles of mastication can also be seen extending anteriorly from the foramen ovale.

IMAGING OF NEUROVASCULAR CONTACT

In patients with medically intractable TGN, imaging is often performed to assess for the presence, type, and degree of neurovascular conflict in the cerebellopontine cistern (**Fig. 4**) and to rule out secondary causes of TGN, including MS as well as benign and malignant neoplasms. For the purposes of this review, the term, *neurovascular conflict*, encompasses the spectrum of findings that may be encountered both on imaging and intraoperatively, ranging in severity from simple contact without nerve displacement or distortion, to severe compression and/or displacement of the nerve, often with associated loss of volume in the nerve root.

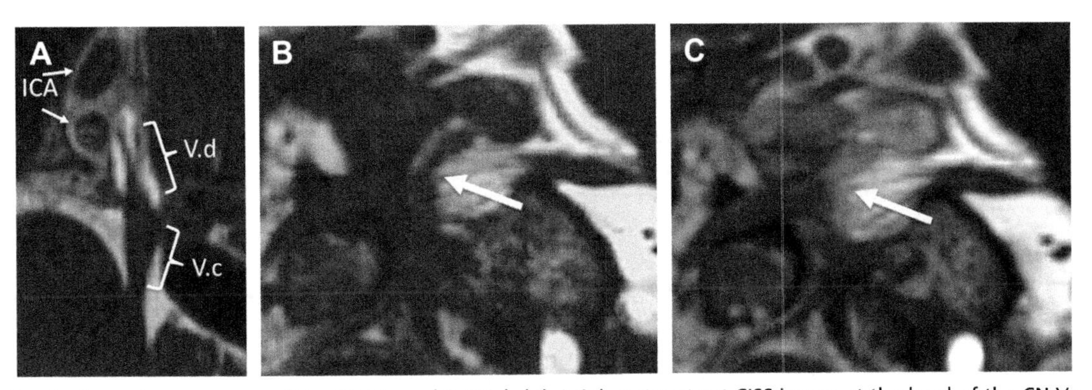

Fig. 1. Normal appearance of the CN V.c and CN V.d. (*A*) Axial postcontrast CISS image at the level of the CN V.c and CN V.d. The internal carotid artery (ICA) is noted medially. (*B*) Precontrast CISS sagittal oblique image of Meckel's cave. Arrow demonstrates normal appearance of gasserian ganglion, which has a crescentic shape along the anterior and inferior margin of Meckel's cave. (*C*) Postcontrast sequence demonstrates normal enhancement of the gasserian ganglion.

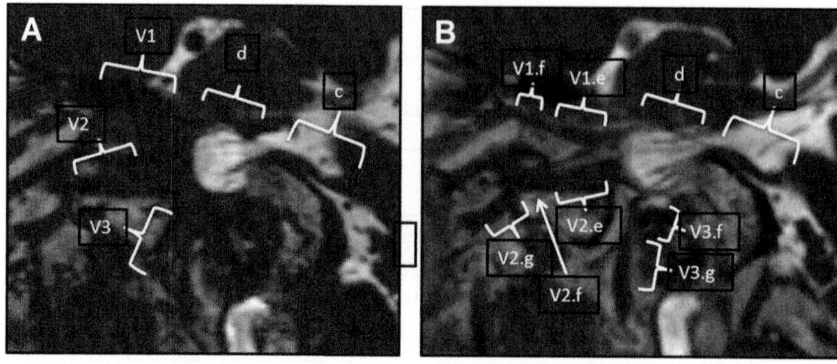

Fig. 2. Normal appearance of CN V without and with contrast. (*A*) Precontrast sagittal oblique CISS centered at Meckel's cave. c, CN V.c. d, CN V.d traverses Meckel's cave and extends to the gasserian ganglion anteriorly. Interdural, foraminal, and extraforaminal segments of V.1, V.2, and V.3 are obscured by cavernous sinus and extensive perineural venous plexus. (*B*) Postcontrast sagittal oblique CISS of CN V at the same level as in (*A*). Interdural (e), foraminal (f), and extraforaminal (g) segments of the respective nerves are labeled. Compared with the unenhanced sequence, V.1–V.3 segments beyond Meckel's cave are now well delineated due to enhancement of the cavernous sinus and perineural venous plexus.

Both the presence and degree of trigeminal root compression have been shown intraoperatively[5–7] and on preoperative imaging[8–10] to be predictive of favorable outcomes after microvascular decompression (MVD). For example, Leal and colleagues[8] showed that 35 of 39 patients (89.7%) with high-grade neurovascular conflict (defined as displacement, distortion, or indentation of the nerve) detected at the time of preoperative imaging were pain-free 2 years after surgery, whereas this was only the case for 6 of 11 (54.5%) patients with no contact or only simple contact detected at the time of preoperative imaging. Duan and colleagues[10] showed that trigeminal root atrophy seen on MRI, defined as decreased cross-sectional area near the root entry zone, was correlated with good surgical outcomes but that the presence of nerve atrophy more distally near the porus trigeminus was associated with poorer outcomes in some of the patients at a median of 13 months after surgery. Thus, preoperative MRI prior to MVD may have significant prognostic implications.

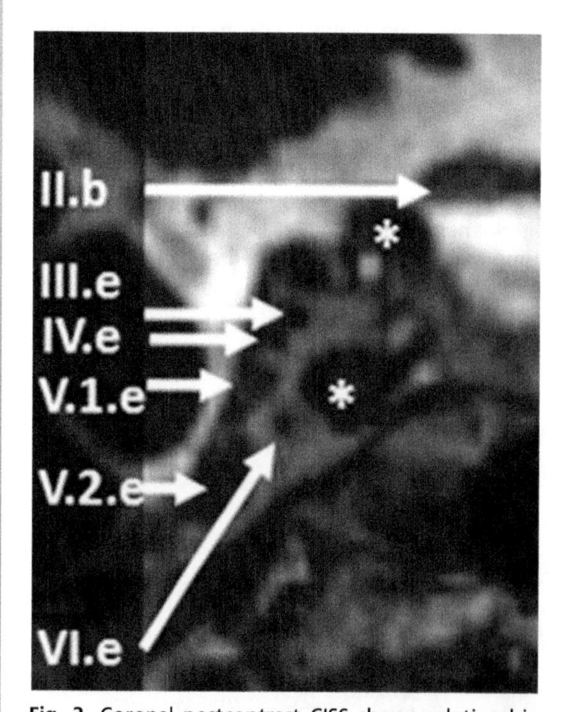

Fig. 3. Coronal postcontrast CISS shows relationship of the interdural CNs in the cavernous sinus. II.b denotes the fascicular segment of the optic nerve (CN II) at the level of the optic chiasm (see Blitz and colleagues[2]). III.e, IV.e, V.1.e, V.2.e, and VI.e denote interdural segments of CN III, CN IV, CN V.1, CN V.2, and CN VI, respectively. The cavernous ICA is seen medially, adjacent to CN VI.e (*asterisks*).

Preoperative imaging gives information about the type of vessel contacting the trigeminal root, the location of contact relative to the apparent origin of the nerve root from the pons, and the surface of the root involved. Traditionally, it has been held that compression syndromes only result when neurovascular conflict occurs at, or near, the root entry zone (also known as the Obersteiner-Redlich zone), which microanatomically constitutes the transition zone between the central and peripheral myelin.[11] The length of centrally myelinated axons along the sensory CN V root is approximately 2 mm to 6 mm.[11] Several imaging studies have shown that arterial contact is more commonly associated with TGN than venous contact[12,13] and that compression in TGN most commonly occurs in the root entry zone,[12,14] although Maarbjerg and colleagues[14] also found that the majority of neurovascular conflict involves arteries close to the apparent origin regardless of

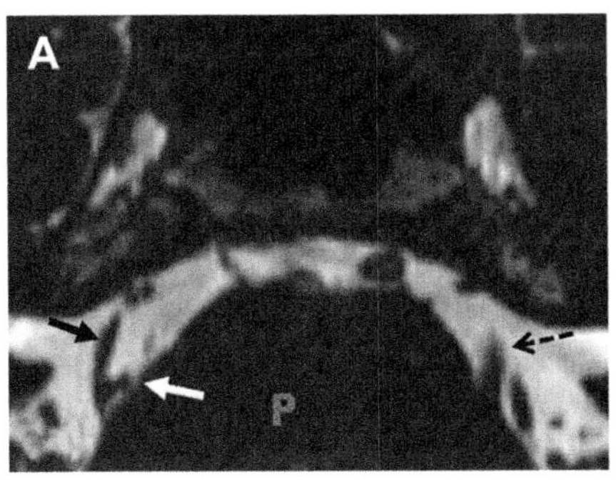

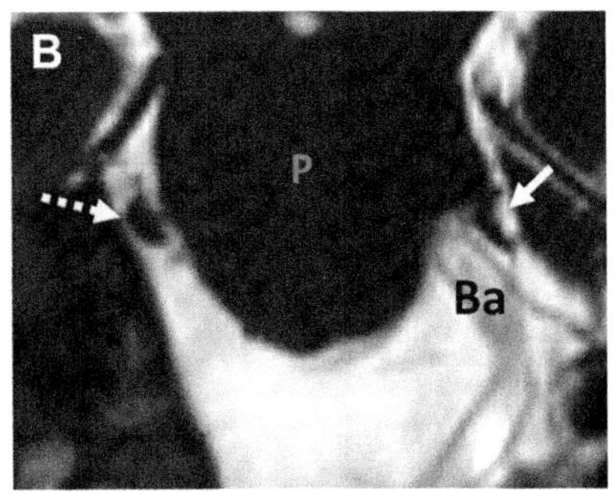

Fig. 4. Examples of neurovascular compression. (*A*) Axial CISS without contrast. The right CN V root (*black solid arrow*) is distorted and compressed by 2 branches of the right superior cerebellar artery (*white arrow*) at the root entry zone near the pons (P). The left CN V root (*interrupted arrow*) is normal. (*B*) Coronal CISS without contrast. The left CN V root (*solid arrow*) is compressed by a tortuous basilar artery (Ba) at the root entry zone near the pons (P). The right trigeminal root (*interrupted arrow*) is normal.

whether it occurs on the symptomatic or asymptomatic side. Sindou and colleagues[5] found no relationship between the location of neurovascular conflict and outcome after surgery, and other investigators have detected neurovascular conflict in the setting of TGN due to venous contact distally along the nerve root near the porus trigeminus.[15] The superior cerebellar artery is the artery most commonly found to contact the trigeminal root, followed by the anterior inferior cerebellar artery,[9,16] and rarely a tortuous basilar artery may come into contact with the nerve root[16] (see **Fig. 4**B).

As previously described, anatomic studies have shown a somatotopic organization to the trigeminal sensory root, with CN V.1 nerve fibers primarily rostral within CN V.c, CN V.2 fibers predominantly medially located in CN V.c, and nerve fibers from the CN V.3 located caudolateral within CN V.c.[3] Zou and colleagues[17] found a similar somatotopic distribution when they correlated preoperative fast imaging employing steady state acquisition (FIESTA) MRI imaging with the distribution of symptoms in TGN patients. Thus, lateral and inferior neurovascular compression corresponded to symptoms predominantly in the V.3 distribution. Compression along the superior and medial surface of the trigeminal root corresponded mostly to symptoms in the V.1 and V.2 distribution.

Preoperative imaging is highly sensitive and specific in detecting neurovascular conflict and shows high agreement with intraoperative findings. For example, in a series with 37 patients with TGN, Zhou and colleagues[17] found that preoperative imaging correctly identified the site of neurovascular compression in 35 of 36 patients with proved intraoperative neurovascular conflict. Importantly, visualization of neurovascular conflict may be difficult intraoperatively, particularly in the setting of distal compression near the porus trigeminus, when a prominent bony ridge along the posterior wall of the petrous temporal bone obscures visualization of CN V, or when the offending vessel is small and located medial and parallel to the nerve.[18–20] Preoperative imaging in those cases may help in surgical planning, for instance, by suggesting the use of an endoscope as an adjunct to the standard operating microscope.[18,19]

Recently, DTI has been used to better understand microstructural tissue changes of the trigeminal root in patients with unilateral TGN. Liu and colleagues[21] measured fractional anisotropy (FA), mean diffusivity, axial diffusivity, and radial diffusivity in the involved CN V roots and found decreased FA and increased radial diffusivity, suggesting demyelination without significant axonal injury as a factor in TGN pathogenesis. Similarly, DeSouza and colleagues[22] found decreased FA in the affected CN V.c and increased mean, axial, and radial diffusivity in the CN V.c on both the affected and unaffected sides in patients with TGN, suggesting nerve root microstructural abnormalities may occur in the trigeminal system as a whole in this patient group. A reversal of these indicators of microstructural abnormalities (decreased FA and increased diffusivity) was found in follow-up imaging in patients after effective MVD, resulting in resolution of facial pain symptoms, but not after ineffective MVD without resolution of symptoms.[23] Thus, in the preoperative assessment of neurovascular conflict, the addition of DTI to high-resolution 3-D cisternogram sequences may provide increased confidence that the observed neurovascular conflict is associated with microstructural tissue changes in the nerve, ostensibly contributing to the patient's symptoms. Future studies are necessary to determine if such imaging findings, in conjunction with high-resolution 3-D cisternogram sequences, can improve the ability to predict which patients are more likely to have successful outcomes after MVD and thus highlight a prognostic role for preoperative imaging in the setting of MVD.

IMAGING OF OTHER CAUSES OF TRIGEMINAL NEURALGIA

TGN in the setting of MS can be due to demyelinating plaques involving the CN V.c, the root entry zone of CN V.b, or CN V.a (**Fig. 5**). Abnormal signal is seen in the root entry zone and CN V.c in approximately 3% to 23% of patients with MS.[24] Another study of 74 patients with MS revealed 5 (6.8%) patients with a lesion at the root entry zone and all had TGN or sensory deficits.[25] Although plaques of the CN V.b or CN V.c can account for symptoms, it is important to keep in mind that neurovascular compression can still occur and cause symptoms in these patients. A study by Broggi and colleagues[26] evaluated 35 patients with MS who underwent MVD for intractable TGN; 26 of the 35 (74%) had demyelinating plaques in the brainstem, with 16 (46%) also having severe neurovascular compression found at the time of surgery. Although outcomes after surgery were not as good as in the case of classical TGN, long-term outcome was still excellent in 39% and good in 14% of patients, suggesting that both central lesions and CN V lesions can play a contributory role in these patients.

As discussed previously, DTI has been used to gain a better understanding of microstructural changes in patients with TGN. Chen and colleagues[27] studied DTI in patients with MS-related TGN and those without MS and found that patients with MS had lower FA in the ipsilateral perilesional central segment of the nerve. The TGN patients without MS, on the other hand, had higher FA in the root entry zone of the CN V ipsilateral to the side of pain, demonstrating that there are differences in the CN V microstructure in TGN and MS-related TGN.[27] Lummel and colleagues[28] demonstrated lower FA values in the CN V.c in patients with MS on both the affected and nonaffected sides compared with controls, indicating more widespread microstructural changes in these patients. Conversely, patients with classical TGN had lower FA values only on the affected side, suggesting a difference in underlying pathogenesis of TGN between MS-related TGN and classical TGN.[28]

When patients with TGN present with sensory loss in a CN V distribution, a possible mass arising along the course of CN V should be suspected. Schwannomas of CN V may occur at any point distal to the transition zone between central and peripheral myelination in CN V.c and can also be associated with TGN. Schwannomas of CN V, which are the second most common intracranial location after those affecting CN VIII, can be seen sporadically or in setting of

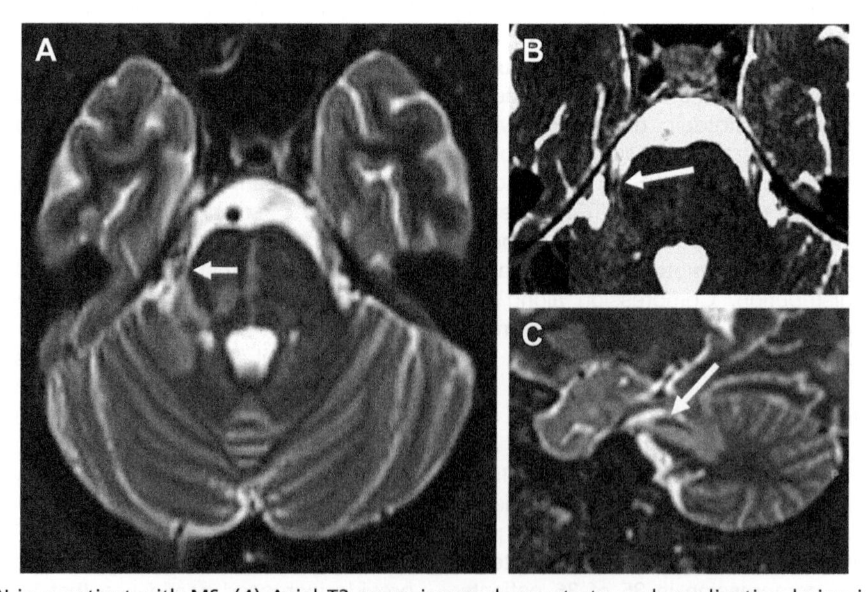

Fig. 5. TGN in a patient with MS. (*A*) Axial T2 space image demonstrates a demyelinating lesion in the right lateral pons near the root entry zone (*arrow*). (*B*) Axial CISS and (*C*) sagittal oblique T2 space images show extension of the demyelinating lesion into the root entry zone of the right CN V (*arrow*).

neurofibromatosis type 2 and rarely undergo malignant transformation. They can appear as small enhancing masses along the course of CN V or as large, cystic, or hemorrhagic masses that can extend through or expand foramina or Meckel's cave. A majority originate within CN V.d at the gasserian ganglion.[29] On CT they present as an isodense mass that can cause smooth expansion and remodeling of foramina through which they pass. On MRI, they are typically isointense or hypointense to gray matter and slightly hyperintense on T2-weighted images and can show solid or heterogeneous enhancement depending on the degree of cystic change or possible hemorrhage present in larger lesions (**Fig. 6**).

Meningiomas of Meckel's cave or of the posterior fossa are another cause of TGN. In a review of 16 patients with meningiomas of Meckel's cave, Delfini and colleagues[30] determined that 15 (93.7%) of those patients presented with trigeminal signs and symptoms. In that review, patients with neuralgia or dysfunction of only CN V were more likely to have isolated Meckel's cave meningiomas compared with those with additional CN symptoms who had extension of meningioma into the cavernous sinus, into the posterior fossa, or into the middle cranial fossa. Meningiomas of Meckel's cave can present as very small or large expansile masses, often isointense to the brain parenchyma on T1-weighted and T2-weighted images with prominent enhancement on postcontrast imaging. They can extend out of Meckel's cave into the cavernous sinus, along the porus trigeminus into the posterior fossa, or to the middle cranial fossa. They can appear hypointense on T1-weighted and T2-weighted sequences when calcifications are present and can be associated with hyperostosis.

Another benign mass that can be associated with TGN is the epidermoid. A review by Furtado and colleagues[31] found 23 reported cases of Meckel's cave epidermoid in the literature, 3 of which had presented with TGN. Epidermoids often present as lesions that are T1 and T2 isointense to cerebrospinal fluid (CSF), slight fluid-attenuated inversion recovery (FLAIR) signal hyperintensity compared with CSF, and with restricted diffusion.

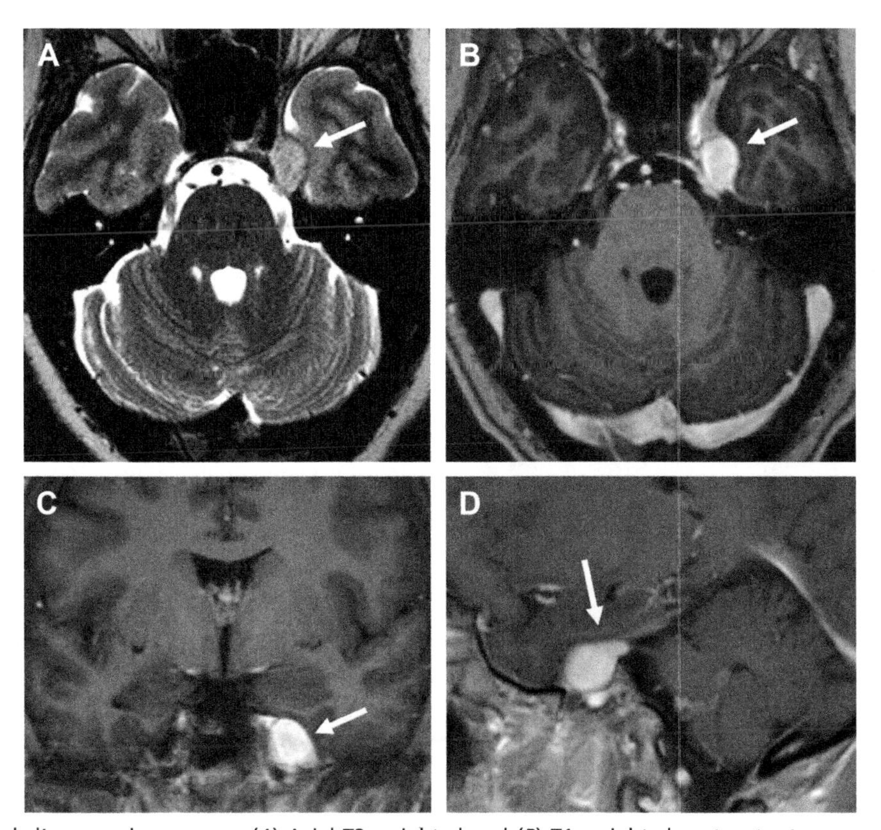

Fig. 6. Meckel's cave schwannoma. (*A*) Axial T2-weighted and (*B*) T1-weighted postcontrast sequences show a well-circumscribed solidly enhancing mass (*arrow*) centered in Meckel's cave on the left that is slightly T2 hyperintense to adjacent gray matter. (*C*) The coronal T1 postcontrast sequence demonstrates mass effect with expansion of Meckel's cave. (*D*) A sagittal oblique image parallel to the course of the CN V.c root nicely shows extension of the mass along the CN V root through the porus trigeminus into the posterior fossa.

Malignant tumor involvement of Meckel's cave can also be associated with TGN, for instance, in the setting of leptomeningeal metastatic disease to the CNs, metastatic involvement of the skull base, or perineural spread of tumor via branches of V.1, V.2, or V.3 (**Fig. 7**). Common causes of perineural spread include melanoma, squamous cell carcinoma, adenoid cystic carcinoma, and lymphoma.[32,33]

POSTOPERATIVE IMAGING AFTER MICROVASCULAR DECOMPRESSION

Imaging in the early postoperative period after MVD is occasionally performed to assess for postoperative complications, which are rare and include meningitis, CSF leak, wound infections, and rarely subdural hematomas.[34] More delayed imaging after MVD is performed to evaluate patients with recurrent symptoms. In this setting, the role of imaging is to assess the relationship of the vessel, nerve, and intervening pad (or polytetrafluoroethylene [Teflon] pledget) or decompressive sling, depending on the type of decompression performed.[34] The pledget or pad is typically hypointense on CISS sequences, does not enhance, and may occasionally become displaced (**Fig. 8**). A Teflon granuloma can occasionally form as a foreign body reaction to the pledget, resulting in mass effect on CN V (**Fig. 9**).[35] Teflon granulomas commonly show enhancement[36] or may calcify.[37] It is important to reassess the CN V.c, looking for other potential sources of neurovascular conflict. The remainder of the course of CN V is also reassessed for any other potential causes of a patient's symptoms, including dense arachnoid adhesions or masses that might be compressing on the nerve. In a series of 12 patients who underwent repeat MVD for recurrent TGN, a vascular loop was found on preoperative imaging and confirmed at surgery in 5 patients (62.5%), a Teflon granuloma was found in 2 patients (25%), and dense arachnoid adhesions were found in 1 patient (12.5%).[35]

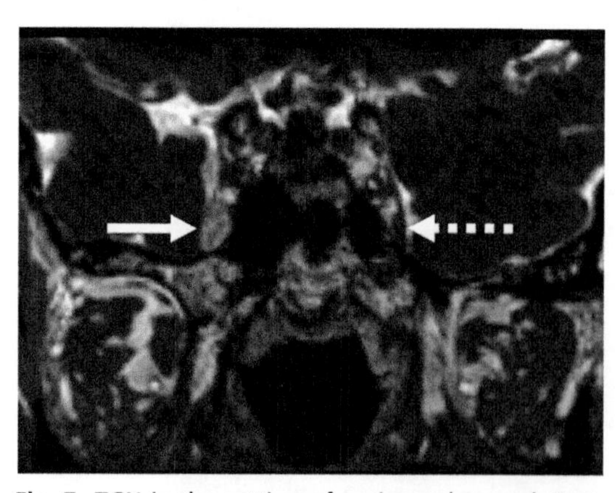

Fig. 7. TGN in the setting of perineural spread. Postcontrast coronal CISS images demonstrate the presence of an enhancing soft tissue mass in the inferior aspect of the anterior right cavernous sinus along the expected route of V.2.e (*white arrow*). Note the normal appearance of the V.2.e nerve on the left side, which is surrounded by enhancing venous contrast in the cavernous sinus but without enhancement of the nerve itself (*dashed arrow*). The right cavernous sinus mass was due to perineural spread from an adenoid cystic carcinoma.

UNDERSTANDING THE PATHOGENESIS OF TRIGEMINAL NEURALGIA THROUGH IMAGING

From the studies described previously using high-resolution 3-D cisternogram and DTI sequences, neurovascular contact, resulting in either demyelination or edema/inflammation of the CN V root, seems to play a contributory role in the pathogenesis of TGN.[21,23] Additional insights into the pathogenesis of TGN have come from MRI studies using tools, like voxel-based morphometry, fMRI, and DTI of brain white matter tracts. fMRI, for example, has been used to better understand the changes in brain activity associated with stimulation of the cutaneous trigger zone in patients with TGN. Moisset and colleagues[38] showed that pain induced by light tactile stimulation of the trigger zone in patients with TGN was associated with pathologic activation of the whole trigeminal nociceptive system, including the spinal trigeminal nucleus and structures involved in pain modulation, suggesting a state of maintained sensitization. After effective treatment, however, activation induced by light tactile stimulation of the trigger zone was confined to primary and secondary somatosensory cortices, suggesting that sensitization of the trigeminal nociceptive system in patients with TGN depends on microstructural abnormalities in CN V.

Using another MRI-based technique, voxel-based morphometry, to quantify volumes of different brain regions, Oberman and colleagues[39] demonstrated widespread gray matter loss in patients with TGN in brain regions well known to be associated with the perception and processing of pain via the trigeminal nociceptive system, including the primary and secondary somatosensory cortices, orbitofrontal cortex, thalamus, and anterior cingulate cortex. The observed changes were thought to reflect a cortical adaptation to chronic pain rather than predisposing to the development of pain itself.

Using similar techniques, DeSouza and colleagues[40] found gray matter alterations in brain

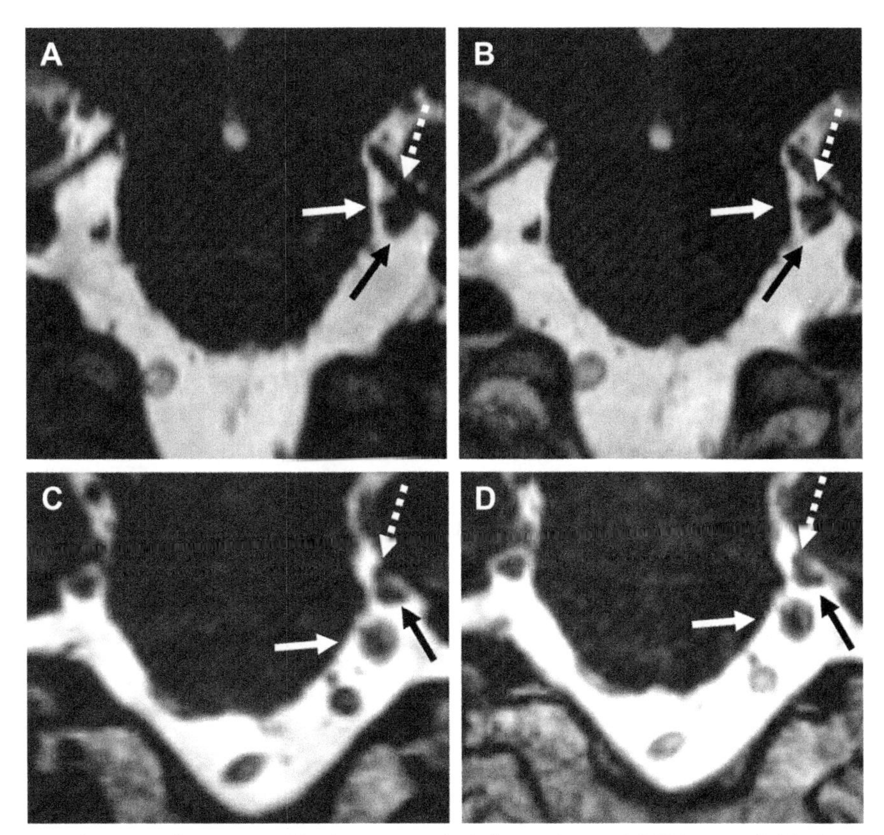

Fig. 8. Postoperative MRI after MVD with placement of pledgets. Coronal CISS images (*A*) before and (*B*) after administration of contrast material demonstrate the expected appearance after pledget placement (*solid white arrow*) between the left CN V root below (*black arrow*) and the superior petrosal vein above (*interrupted white arrow*). Coronal CISS images (*C*) before and (*D*) after contrast administration demonstrate an unexpected gap of CSF between the pledget (*solid white arrow*) and the left CN V root (*black arrow*), which is contacted by a branch of the superior cerebellar artery from above (*interrupted white arrow*). Note the lack of enhancement of the pledget, which differentiates it from a Teflon granuloma, which typically demonstrates postcontrast enhancement.

regions that contribute to pain perception, pain modulation, and motor function. Specifically, they found increased gray matter volume in the sensory thalamus, amygdala, periaqueductal gray, and basal ganglia compared with healthy controls. Patients also had greater cortical thickness in the contralateral primary somatosensory cortex and frontal pole compared with controls but decreased cortical thickness in the pregenual anterior cingulate cortex, the insula, and the orbitofrontal cortex. No relationship was found between the gray matter abnormalities and TGN pain duration. In a follow-up study, DeSouza and colleagues[23] found that after effective surgical intervention resulting in resolution of symptoms, there was reversal of the decreased gray matter thickness in the ipsilateral ventral anterior insula, which was interpreted as likely related to decreased nociceptive input from the trigeminal afferents to the CNS. The other gray matter regions, however, showed no reversal after successful surgical intervention. The cause for this is unclear, although one possibility is the short duration (2–6 months) that was chosen between the surgical intervention and imaging. Also unclear is how these gray matter alterations in general play into the pathogenesis of TGN. Possibilities include that they represent a response to chronic increased nociceptive input to the brain as well as learned compensatory motor behaviors, although in that case it might have been expected that more or all of the gray matter alterations would have normalized after effective surgical treatment. Alternatively, some individuals may be more susceptible to developing chronic pain because of preexisting gray matter abnormalities. Longer-term follow-up imaging in patients after effective surgery might help distinguish between these possibilities.

Using tract-based spatial statistics on DTI data, DeSouza and colleagues[22] found widespread regions of brain white matter abnormalities in patients with TGN, with lower FA and higher radial and mean diffusivity compared with healthy

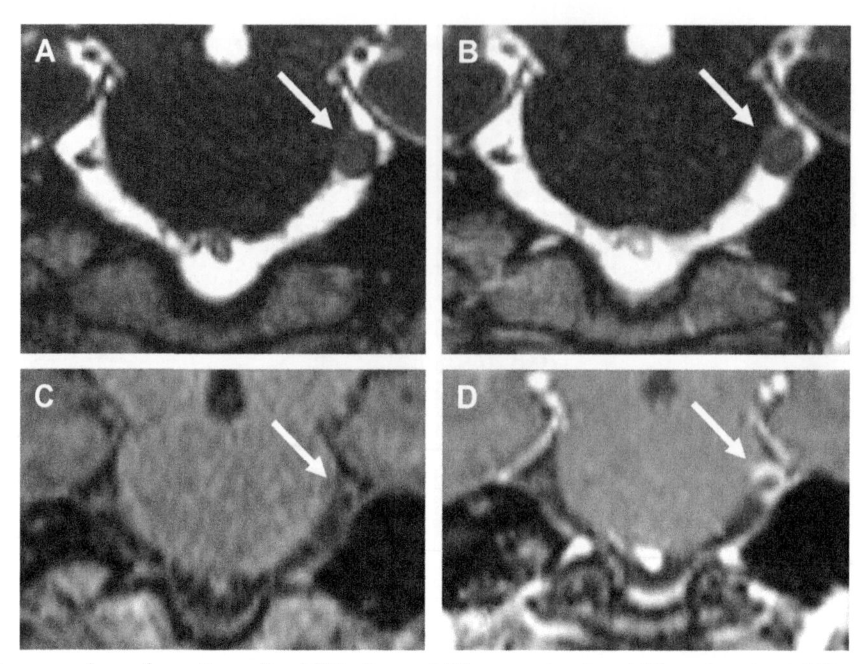

Fig. 9. Teflon granuloma formation after MVD. Coronal (*A*) precontrast and (*B*) postcontrast CISS as well as (*C*) precontrast and (*D*) postcontrast VIBE images show a well-circumscribed enhancing soft tissue lesion (*arrow*) with central hypoenhancement, which is not clearly separable from the left CN V root. This was presumed to represent a Teflon granuloma.

controls. Regions most affected were the corpus callosum, the cingulum, the posterior corona radiata, and the superior longitudinal fasciculus. These white matter tracts connect brain regions known to participate in the multidimensional experience of pain, attention, and motor function and may play a contributory role in the symptoms of TGN pain and/or in the compensatory pain-avoiding motor behaviors seen in these patients. The DTI changes in brain white matter may result from decreased fiber organization, including more axonal sprouting/branching, more crossing fibers, or larger axons. Another possibility includes central sensitization related to prolonged nociceptive input to the brain, which can result in central neuroinflammation and edema. Similar to the gray matter changes described previously, it is still unclear whether these white matter changes are a result of prolonged nociceptive input or represent an underlying predisposing condition.

SUMMARY

Advanced imaging in TGN continues to evolve. High-resolution isotropic MRI is now routinely performed and allows imaging of nearly the entire course of CN V in exquisite anatomic detail. Presurgical evaluation in patients with medically intractable TGN allows assessment for the presence, type, and degree of neurovascular conflict in the cerebellopontine cistern and also allows for assessment of secondary causes of TGN, including MS, as well as benign and malignant neoplasms. Postoperative imaging in the setting of recurrent pain after MVD allows assessment of the relationship of the nerve, vessel, and interposed pad, pledget, or sling, depending on method of decompression, and allows reassessment for additional sources of neurovascular conflict or masses compressing on the nerve, including Teflon granulomas and dense arachnoid adhesions. Advanced MRI imaging techniques, like DTI, voxel-based morphometry, and fMRI, are providing insight into the pathogenesis of TGN. Future studies linking presurgical imaging to intraoperative findings and clinical outcomes data will help continue to define the role of imaging in preoperative planning and clinical management decisions.

REFERENCES

1. Blitz A, Choudhri A, Chonka Z, et al. Anatomic considerations, nomenclature, and advanced cross-sectional imaging techniques for visualization of the cranial nerve segments by MR imaging. Neuroimaging Clin N Am 2014;24(1):1–15.
2. Blitz A, Macedo L, Chonka Z, et al. High-resolution CISS MR imaging with and without contrast for

evaluation of the upper cranial nerves. Neuroimaging Clin N Am 2014;24(1):17–34.
3. Gudmundsson K, Rhoton AL Jr, Rushton JG. Detailed anatomy of the intracranial portion of the trigeminal nerve. J Neurosurg 1971;35(5):592–600.
4. Rodella LF, Buffoli B, Labanca M, et al. A review of the mandibular and maxillary nerve supplies and their clinical relevance. Arch Oral Biol 2012;57(4):323–34.
5. Sindou M, Leston J, Decullier E, et al. Microvascular decompression for primary trigeminal neuralgia: long-term effectiveness and prognostic factors of 362 consecutive patients with clear-cut neurovascular conflicts who underwent pure decompression. J Neurosurg 2007;107(6):1144–53.
6. Hamlyn PJ. Neurovascular relationships in the posterior cranial fossa, with special reference to trigeminal neuralgia. 2. Neurovascular compression of the trigeminal nerve in cadaveric controls and patients with trigeminal neuralgia: quantification and influence of method. Clin Anat 1997;10(6):380–8.
7. Szapiro J Jr, Sindou M, Szapiro J. Prognostic factors in microvascular decompression for trigeminal neuralgia. Neurosurgery 1985;17(6):920–9.
8. Leal PR, Barbier C, Hermier M, et al. Atrophic changes in the trigeminal nerves of patients with trigeminal neuralgia due to neurovascular compression and their association with the severity of compression and clinical outcomes. J Neurosurg 2014;120(6):1484–95.
9. Han-Bing S, Wei-Guo Z, Jun Z, et al. Predicting the outcome of microvascular decompression for trigeminal neuralgia using magnetic resonance tomographic angiography. J Neuroimaging 2010;20(4):345–9.
10. Duan Y, Sweet J, Munyon C, et al. Degree of distal trigeminal nerve atrophy predicts outcome after microvascular decompression for type 1a trigeminal neuralgia. J Neurosurg 2015;17:1–7.
11. Yousry I, Moriggl B, Holtmannspoetter M, et al. Detailed anatomy of the motor and sensory roots of the trigeminal nerve and their neurovascular relationships: a magnetic resonance imaging study. J Neurosurg 2004;101(3):427–34.
12. Antonini G, Di Pasquale A, Cruccu G, et al. Magnetic resonance imaging contribution for diagnosing symptomatic neurovascular contact in classical trigeminal neuralgia: a blinded case-control study and meta-analysis. Pain 2014;155(8):1464–71.
13. Leal PR, Hermier M, Souza MA, et al. Visualization of vascular compression of the trigeminal nerve with high-resolution 3T MRI: a prospective study comparing preoperative imaging analysis to surgical findings in 40 consecutive patients who underwent microvascular decompression for trigeminal neuralgia. Neurosurgery 2011;69(1):15–25.
14. Maarbjerg S, Wolfram F, Gozalov A, et al. Significance of neurovascular contact in classical trigeminal neuralgia. Brain 2015;138(Pt 2):311–9.
15. Hong W, Zheng X, Wu Z, et al. Clinical features and surgical treatment of trigeminal neuralgia caused solely by venous compression. Acta Neurochir (Wien) 2011;153(5):1037–42.
16. Leal PR, Hermier M, Froment JC, et al. Preoperative demonstration of the neurovascular compression characteristics with special emphasis on the degree of compression, using high-resolution magnetic resonance imaging: a prospective study, with comparison to surgical findings, in 100 consecutive patients who underwent microvascular decompression for trigeminal neuralgia. Acta Neurochir (Wien) 2010;152(5):817–25.
17. Zhou Q, Liu ZL, Qu CC, et al. Preoperative demonstration of neurovascular relationship in trigeminal neuralgia by using 3D FIESTA sequence. Magn Reson Imaging 2012;30(5):666–71.
18. Broggi M, Acerbi F, Ferroli P, et al. Microvascular decompression for neurovascular conflicts in the cerebello-pontine angle: which role for endoscopy? Acta Neurochir (Wien) 2013;155(9):1709–16.
19. Sandell T, Ringstad GA, Eide PK. Usefulness of the endoscope in microvascular decompression for trigeminal neuralgia and MRI-based prediction of the need for endoscopy. Acta Neurochir (Wien) 2014;156(10):1901–9.
20. Bohman LE, Pierce J, Stephen JH, et al. Fully endoscopic microvascular decompression for trigeminal neuralgia: technique review and early outcomes. Neurosurg Focus 2014;37(4):E18.
21. Liu Y, Li J, Butzkueven H, et al. Microstructural abnormalities in the trigeminal nerves of patients with trigeminal neuralgia revealed by multiple diffusion metrics. Eur J Radiol 2013;82(5):783–6.
22. DeSouza DD, Hodaie M, Davis KD. Abnormal trigeminal nerve microstructure and brain white matter in idiopathic trigeminal neuralgia. Pain 2014;155(1):37–44.
23. DeSouza DD, Davis KD, Hodaie M. Reversal of insular and microstructural nerve abnormalities following effective surgical treatment for trigeminal neuralgia. Pain 2015;156(6):1112–23.
24. Mills RJ, Young CA, Smith ET. Central trigeminal involvement in multiple sclerosis using high-resolution MRI at 3T. Br J Radiol 2010;83(990):493–8.
25. Nakashima I, Fujihara K, Kimpara T, et al. Linear pontine trigeminal root lesions in multiple sclerosis: clinical and magnetic resonance imaging studies in 5 cases. Arch Neurol 2001;58(1):101–4.
26. Broggi G, Ferroli P, Franzini A, et al. Operative findings and outcomes of microvascular decompression for trigeminal neuralgia in 35 patients affected by multiple sclerosis. Neurosurgery 2004;55(4):830–8.

27. Chen DQ, DeSouza DD, Hayes DJ, et al. Diffusivity signatures characterize trigeminal neuralgia associated with multipe sclerosis. Mult Scler 2016;22(1):51–63.
28. Lummel N, Mehrkens JH, Linn J, et al. Diffusion tensor imaging of the trigeminal nerve in patients with trigeminal neuralgia due to multiple sclerosis. Neuroradiology 2015;57(3):259–67.
29. Majoie CB, Verbeeten B Jr, Dol JA, et al. Trigeminal neuropathy: evaluation with MR imaging. Radiographics 1995;15(4):795–811.
30. Delfini R, Innocenzi G, Ciappetta P, et al. Meningiomas of meckel's cave. Neurosurgery 1992;31(6):1000–6.
31. Furtado SV, Hegde AS. Tigeminal neuralgia due to a small meckel's cave epidermoid tumor: surgery using an extradural corridor. Skull Base 2009;19(5):353–7.
32. Chang PC, Fischbein NJ, McCalmont TH, et al. Perineural spread of malignant melanoma of the head and neck: clinical and imaging features. AJNR Am J Neuroradiol 2004;25:5–11.
33. Parker GD, Harnsberger HR. Clinical-radiologic issues in perineural tumor spread of malignant diseases of the extracranial head and neck. Radiographics 1991;11(3):383–99.
34. Zakrzewska JM. CoakhamHB. Microvascular decompression for trigeminal neuralgia: update. Curr Opin Neurol 2012;25(3):296–301.
35. Gu W, Zhao W. Microvascular decompression for recurrent trigeminal neuralgia. J Clin Neurosci 2014;21(9):1549–53.
36. Capelle HH, Brandis A, Tschan CA, et al. Treatment of recurrent trigeminal neuralgia due to Teflon granuloma.
37. Sharma G, Chaturvdi A, Kapoor D. Teflon granuloma: A rare cause of recurrent trigeminal neuralgia. Neurol India 2015;63(5):803–4.
38. Moisset X, Villain N, Ducreux D, et al. Functional brain imaging of trigeminal neuralgia. Eur J Pain 2011;15(2):124–31.
39. Obermann M, Rodriguez-Raecke R. Gray matter volume reduction reflects chronic pain in trigeminal neuralgia. Neuroimage 2013;74:352–8.
40. Desouza DD, Moayedi M, Chen DQ, et al. Sensorimotor and pain modulation brain abnormalities in trigeminal neuralgia: A paroxysmal, sensory-triggered neuropathic pain. PLoS One 2013;8(6):e66340.

Measurement of Trigeminal Neuralgia Pain

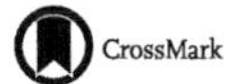

Penn Facial Pain Scale

ohn Y.K. Lee, MD, MSCE

KEYWORDS

- Barrow Neurological Institute Pain Intensity Score • Brief pain inventory • McGill Pain Questionnaire
- Numeric rating scale • Patient-reported outcomes • Trigeminal neuralgia • Visual analog scale
- Penn Facial Pain Scale

KEY POINTS

- The subjective and multidimensional quality of pain makes it challenging to study and emphasizes that a patient's perception of pain should be accepted as the most valid reporting.
- Patient-reported outcome (PRO) tools capture patient's pain ratings in a structured and reproducible format that also allows patients to evaluate their current condition and treatment.
- The Penn Facial Pain Scale is a multidimensional pain scale that assesses facial pain intensity and facial pain interference with activities of daily living and facial-specific activities.
- A composite questionnaire that combines multiple PROs should address the six domains of the Initiative on Methods, Measurement, and Pain Assessment in Clinical trials.

NTRODUCTION

Pain is a personal experience—it is impossible for a person to understand or experience another person's pain. Even patients who experience the same pain stimuli or interventions have wide variability of their pain ratings.[1] Pain is also more than just a sensory experience; it has physical, emotional, and social implications. The subjective and multidimensional quality of pain makes it challenging to study and emphasizes that a patient's perception of pain should be accepted as the most valid reporting.[2–4] Patient-reported outcome (PRO) tools are an excellent way to capture those pain ratings because they provide a structured and reproducible format that also allows patients to evaluate their current health condition and treatment.[5] PROs are instrumental for measuring pain because patients are the only source of information, clinical assessments may not parallel a patient's actual pain or disability, and patients should be the ones to decide whether or not their clinical change is actually meaningful.[5,6]

The purpose of this article is to provide an overview of different PROs that can be used to measure pain and outcomes in trigeminal neuralgia (TN). There are several scales that can be used to measure pain, and readers are encouraged to choose the most appropriate outcome measure. Although there are several different PROs that can be used, the main issue with evaluating treatment response and efficacy is the lack of a consensus on which scale to use and defined criteria for outcomes.[1] With the availability of many treatment options for TN, which range from conservative pharmacotherapy to neurosurgical intervention with Gamma Knife radiosurgery (RS), percutaneous stereotactic radiofrequency lesioning (RFL), and microvascular decompression (MVD), it is necessary to develop a uniform process of measuring pain in TN to compare the outcomes of different treatments. The PROs

Disclosure Statement: None.
Department of Neurosurgery, University of Pennsylvania, 235 S. 8th Street, Philadelphia, PA 19107, USA
E-mail address: john.lee3@uphs.upenn.edu

Neurosurg Clin N Am 27 (2016) 327–336
http://dx.doi.org/10.1016/j.nec.2016.02.003

discussed in this article have been evaluated for practicality, applicability, comprehensiveness, reliability, validity, and sensitivity to measuring TN pain in addition to adherence to the six domains outlined by the Initiative on Methods, Measurement, and Pain Assessment in Clinical Trials (IMMPACT) (**Tables 1** and **2**).

REVIEW OF PAIN SCALES AND PATIENT-REPORTED OUTCOME MEASURES

Visual Analog Scale

Format

The visual analog scale (VAS) is a simple, 1-dimensional (1-D) scale that measures pain intensity (**Fig. 1**). It is a 10-cm horizontal line with word anchors on either end. The word anchors can be changed to represent different dimensions of pain.[7] The anchors most commonly used in pain studies are "no pain" and "worst possible pain." Specific points along the line can be labeled with intensity-denoting adjectives or numbers; the scale is then referred to as a graphic rating scale. Patients are asked to mark the point on the line that represents the intensity of their pain. The VAS score is determined by measuring the distance in millimeters from the left hand side of the line to the point where the patient marked the line. The scale requires special materials (pen and paper), vision, and dexterity.

Evaluation

The VAS has been widely used and is well validated, reliable, and internally consistent when used to measure the intensity of pain.[7,8] It has been used in several studies evaluating different treatments of TN, including pharmacotherapy, Gamma Knife RS, RFL, and MVD.[9–12] The VAS is comprehensive and also a form of cross-modality matching because it uses a direct scaling technique. Thus, results can be presented as a ratio rather than as an interval, which allows for more meaningful statements regarding pain magnitude.[7,13] For example, when a group of patients have shown a change in pain intensity of 80 to 40, their pain has been reduced by half.

The major critique of the VAS is that a majority of patients have difficulty discerning pain intensity, distress caused by pain, and how pain affects their quality of life. Scores on the VAS are often affected by changes in functional status, emotional effects, physical limitations, and pain-associated symptoms.[14] Therefore, VAS scores may not singularly represent pain intensity; they may actually be more representative of pain intensity and distress caused by the pain.[14] Although the VAS score can be affected by many different aspects of pain, it only specifically addresses the pain domain from the IMMPACT recommendations. Another limitation of the VAS is its impracticality—it requires special materials (paper form and pen) and dexterity. Therefore, the scale can only be administered in person or mailed, and it excludes populations with limited dexterity and vision, such as the geriatric population. It cannot be administered over the telephone because it is a graphic measure of pain, but it does provide a continuous outcome variable, which can be useful for evaluation.

Numeric Rating Scale for Pain Intensity

Format

The numeric rating scale for pain intensity (NRS-PI) is a 1-D scale used to measure pain intensity (**Fig. 2**). It is a series of numbers ranging from

Table 1
Evaluation and selection criteria for outcome measures

Criteria	Description
Applicable	Content and emphasis of the measure are relevant and disease-specific
Practical	Minimal respondent and administrative burden
Comprehensive	Addresses multidimensional components of disease burden (physical, psychosocial, etc.)
Reliable	Acceptable test-retest, inter-rater, and internal consistency reliability
Valid	Criterion: accuracy of the measure compared with gold standard Construct: ability to measure what it intends to measure Content: measurement is representative of the construct it is intended to measure
Sensitive	Correctly identify patients with disease and ability to detect differences that would be considered significant

Adapted from Deyo RA. Measuring functional outcomes in therapeutic trials for chronic disease. Control Clin Trials 1984;5(3):223–40; and Deyo RA, Centor RM. Assessing the responsiveness of functional scales to clinical change: an analogy to diagnostic test performance. J Chronic Dis 1986;39:897–906.

Table 2
Initiative on methods, measurement, and pain assessment in clinical trials: recommendations for core outcome measures

Domain	Recommended Measure
Pain	11-Point (0–10) numeric rating scale (preferred) or categorical ratings (eg, none mild, moderate, severe) of pain intensity
Physical functioning	Multidimensional Pain Inventory Interference Scale Brief Pain Inventory
Emotional functioning	Beck Depression Inventory Profile of Mood States
Global improvement or satisfaction	Patient Global Impression of Change
Symptoms and adverse events	Spontaneous reporting of symptoms and adverse events with open-ended prompts
Participant disposition	Participant recruitment and progress information

Adapted from Dworkin RH, Turk DC, Wyrwich KW, et al. Interpreting the clinical importance of treatment outcomes in chronic pain clinical trials: IMMPACT recommendations. J Pain 2008;9:105–21; and Dworkin R, Farrar J. Research design issues in pain clinical trials. Neurology 2005;65(12) Suppl 4:S1–2. Available at: http://www.neurology.org/content/65/12_suppl_4/S1.short.

0 to 10 or 0 to 100, where the 2 respective endpoints are "no pain" and "worst possible pain." Patients are asked to rate their pain at the time of completing the scale by selecting the number that best represents their level of pain. There are also variations of the scale that ask patients to rate different categories and intensities of their pain, such as their pain at its "worst," "least," "average," and "right now." The NRS-PI can be administered in person or over the telephone; it does not require special materials, vision, or dexterity.

Evaluation

The NRS has been well validated, has demonstrated positive correlation with different measures of pain, and has shown sensitivity to treatments known to improve pain intensity.[4,15,16] The NRS is also a practical tool and has been widely used in several chronic pain trials. Unlike the VAS, the scale does not require special materials, the scoring is intuitive, and it can be administered verbally or over the telephone. The NRS and the VAS have been compared in several studies, and although both scales have proved validity and responsiveness, the intuitive nature of the NRS and its ability to be administered both in person and over the telephone give it an advantage over the VAS.[4,17,18]

One major weakness of the NRS is its lack of ratio qualities,[8] meaning that when a group of patients has shown a change in pain intensity of 8 to 4, it does not necessarily mean that their pain was been reduced by half. The scale is also 1-D and only addresses the pain domain from the IMMPACT recommendations.

Barrow Neurological Institute Pain Intensity Score

Format

The Barrow Neurological Institute Pain Intensity Score (BNI-PS) is a composite pain scale that measures pain intensity with a score (**Table 3**). This scale is complicated because it requires an assessment of 3 distinct outcome measures and only some of the possible combinations are listed as choices for the BNI-PS. The first outcome domain is pain intensity defined into 4 discrete choices: none, occasional, some, and severe. The second outcome domain is the use of medications categorized as either yes or no response. The third domain is a subjective assessment by the patient or the practitioner (not specified in the design) as to whether the pain is controlled and categorized as either a yes or no response. The scale has typically been administered on paper, but it has the ability of being completed verbally in person or over the telephone.

Fig. 1. VAS.

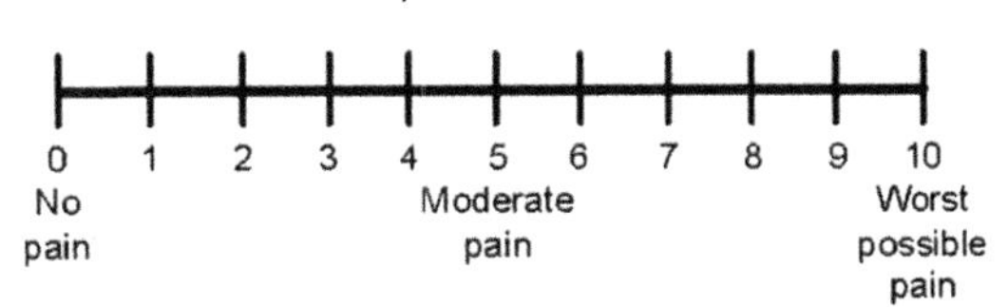

Fig. 2. The 0 to 10 numeric rating scale.

Table 3
Barrow Neurological Institute Pain Intensity Score

Score	
I	No trigeminal pain, no medication
II	Occasional pain, not requiring medication
III	Some pain, adequately controlled with medication
IV	Some pain, not adequately controlled with medication
V	Severe pain/no pain relief

Adapted from Rogers CL, Shetter AG, Fiedler JA, et al. Gamma knife radiosurgery for trigeminal neuralgia: the initial experience of The Barrow Neurological Institute. Int J Radiat Oncol Biol Phys 2000;47:1015; with permission.

Evaluation

The BNI-PS was initially developed and published by the Barrow Neurological Institute for a study that evaluated outcomes after Gamma Knife RS.[19] It is an easy-to-use scale that seems to have high face validity. It can be administered in person or over the telephone, and it does not require special materials. Since the publication of the initial study, several researchers have used the scale to determine outcomes after RS.[19–21]

The major advantage of the BNI-PS is that it was specifically created for measuring treatment outcomes in TN; however, there are many significant limitations. First, the scale itself is a composite of 3 outcome domains. Based on the 3 variables of interest, there are 16 possible answers, but only 5 are included in the actual BNI-PS. There seems not to be any validated reason as to why only 5 of the possible 16 permutations of level of pain severity, the need for medication, and pain control were chosen for the actual score. For example, one possible outcome is that the individual experiences "no pain" but does require medications. This outcome cannot be selected from the BNI-PS. The psychometric properties of the BNI-PS have not been tested; therefore, the validity and reliability of the scale have not been verified. Similarly, its ratio properties have not been established. Is a change from 4 to 2 a 50% improvement? Does it represent a patient-specific clinically important difference?

In addition, only the pain and patient disposition domains of the IMMPACT recommendations were addressed. The patient disposition criterion is only partially determined by asking patients whether they require medication for pain control.

McGill Pain Questionnaire

Format

The McGill Pain Questionnaire (MPQ) is a multidimensional scale that includes 20 subclasses of words used to describe pain. The subclasses are derived from 4 major classes of the pain experience: (1) sensory qualities (temporal, spatial, pressure, and thermal properties), (2) affective qualities (tension, fear, and autonomic properties), (3) evaluative words used to describe the intensity of the pain, and (4) a miscellaneous class.[4] Patients are instructed to select only the words that describe their pain. After the descriptor words have been selected, 3 indices are obtained from the patient: (1) pain rating index, where patients are asked to rank the words within each subclass, and a total score is calculated from those selections; (2) the total number of words selected from the entire questionnaire; and (3) the present pain intensity (PPI), where patients are instructed to rate their pain on a scale from 0 to 5 at the time of completing the questionnaire. This PRO can be administered verbally or as a paper form.

The Short-Form MPQ (SF-MPQ) was designed for use in time-limited scenarios, such as research.[4] The questionnaire consists of 15 words from the sensory and affective categories of the MPQ, the PPI, and the VAS. Patients are asked to rank the 15 descriptor words with an intensity score that ranges from 0 to 3 (0 = "none," 1 = "mild," 2 = "moderate," and 3 = "severe").

Evaluation

The MPQ has been used in hundreds of studies on pain and has been translated into 20 languages. The questionnaire has proved validity, reliability, and consistency.[4,22–24] The PRO has been used in studies of TN and has shown discriminative ability to differentiate classic TN pain from atypical facial pain.[25,26] The inclusion of words, such as dull pain, aching pain, and continuous pain, in the questionnaire helps identify patients with atypical facial pain. That information can aid neurosurgeons when deciding on treatment options because patients with atypical facial pain have had poor outcomes after surgery.[4,27] The MPQ has also been used in composite questionnaires that were developed for evaluating TN outcomes.[10,28]

The MPQ has many advantages. It is practical because it can be administered either as a paper form or over the telephone. In addition, the 3-factor structure of the PRO (sensory, affective, and evaluative) addresses the pain, emotional functioning, and symptom domains of the IMMPACT recommendations. The major downside of the

MPQ is the complexity of the vocabulary needed to understand the MPQ.

Penn Facial Pain Scale

Format

The Penn Facial Pain Scale (PFPS) is a multidimensional pain scale that assesses facial pain intensity and facial pain interference with activities of daily living and facial-specific activities (**Fig. 3**). It was originally called the BPI-Facial, but its name has been changed to the PFPS. This scale incorporates the original Brief Pain Inventory and adds an additional 7 facial interference items tested for reliability and validity. Pain intensity is measured using the NRS—patients are asked to rate their pain intensity at its worst, least, average, and current level of pain. Patients are also asked to rate how their pain interferes with general activities (general activity, mood, walking ability, normal work, relationships with other people, sleep, and enjoyment of life) and facial-specific activities (eating a meal, touching one's face, brushing or flossing one's teeth, smiling or laughing, talking, opening one's mouth widely, and eating hard food like apples). The questionnaire is typically administered on paper and over the telephone.

Evaluation

The PFPS includes the Brief Pain Inventory, which is a scale originally developed by the Pain Research Group of the World Health Organization Collaborating Centre for Symptom Evaluation in Cancer Care to measure pain in cancer patients. Numerous studies have proved that the BPI is both valid and reliable for measuring pain in cancer patients, disabled patients, and patients with chronic nonmalignant pain.[29–32] Lee and colleagues included the BPI and expanded it to include 7 additional items specific to facial activities to specifically evaluate facial pain disorders. The 7 items were created after reviewing TN literature and consulting neurosurgical experts and patients with facial pain disorders.[33]

The psychometric properties of the PRO were studied and demonstrated that the scale is highly reliable based on its excellent factor analysis properties (internal consistency). The scale also demonstrated face and content validity—the scale was evaluated by a group of TN experts, including 3 neurosurgeons, to ensure that it addressed the desired qualities and sampled relevant content.[34] Construct validity was tested with factor analysis of the 3 domains measured by the PFPS and the scale's ability to differentiate between atypical facial pain and classic TN.[34]

There are many advantages to using the PFPS. The scale is applicable to TN because there are 7 disease-specific questions that pertain to facial pain syndromes. The scale is also practical because it can be administered verbally or on paper. It is also comprehensive because it addresses the multidimensional quality of pain. The limitation of the scale is that it only addresses the pain and physical functioning domains from the IMMPACT recommendations.

RECOMMENDATIONS FOR DEVELOPING A PAIN SCALE

Although at least 5 outcome tools for measurement of pain exist and can be used to measure TN pain, it is unfortunately rare to see them used in the neurosurgical, neurologic, and dental literature. Both the limited use of PROs and the lack of uniformity in measuring pain and response to treatments have made it difficult to establish a clear-cut standard for TN patient outcomes. If there were 1 universally used scale with a set standard for the TN population, data from various studies could be aggregated and treatments compared objectively, research protocols could be developed, and large-scale literature reviews could be conducted.[6,35] These issues are evident in a literature review of 222 studies that evaluated the quality of reporting of TN surgical outcomes. Only 28 studies could be used to evaluate outcomes because they had actuarial analysis, and only 32 studies used patient questionnaires or telephone interviews.[28]

The lack of adoption of a single standard PRO for TN has hindered the comparison of treatments and patient outcomes. It is admittedly difficult to evaluate chronic pain because it is complex—it is a multifaceted interplay of physiology and patient expectations, mood, coping mechanisms, level of function, and sociocultural context.[35] There are several factors to consider when deciding on which uniform scale to use. Deyo reviewed numerous quality-of-life indices and scales and found that measurement tools should have the following qualities: applicability, practicality, comprehensiveness, reliability, validity, and sensitivity to the disease (see **Table 1**).[36,37] In addition, the Initiative on Methods, Measurement, and Pain Assessment in Clinical Trials (IMMPACT) identified 6 core outcome domains that should be considered when developing a clinical trial that is focused on the efficacy and effectiveness of a treatment. The 6 core domains are (1) pain, (2) physical functioning, (3) emotional functioning, (4) participant ratings of global improvement, (5) symptoms and adverse events, and (6) participant disposition

Circle the ONE number that describes how, during the past week, pain has interfered with your:

1. General Activity

   0 1 2 3 4 5 6 7 8 9 10

   Does not interfere — Completely interferes

2. Mood

   0 1 2 3 4 5 6 7 8 9 10

   Does not interfere — Completely interferes

3. Walking Ability

   0 1 2 3 4 5 6 7 8 9 10

   Does not interfere — Completely interferes

4. Normal Work (includes both work outside the home and housework)

   0 1 2 3 4 5 6 7 8 9 10

   Does not interfere — Completely interferes

5. Relations with other people

   0 1 2 3 4 5 6 7 8 9 10

   Does not interfere — Completely interferes

6. Sleep

   0 1 2 3 4 5 6 7 8 9 10

   Does not interfere — Completely interferes

7. Enjoyment of life

   0 1 2 3 4 5 6 7 8 9 10

   Does not interfere — Completely interferes

---

8. Eating a meal

   0 1 2 3 4 5 6 7 8 9 10

   Does not interfere — Completely interferes

9. Touching your face (including grooming)

   0 1 2 3 4 5 6 7 8 9 10

   Does not interfere — Completely interferes

10. Brushing or flossing your teeth

    0 1 2 3 4 5 6 7 8 9 10

    Does not interfere — Completely interferes

11. Smiling or laughing

    0 1 2 3 4 5 6 7 8 9 10

    Does not interfere — Completely interferes

12. Talking

    0 1 2 3 4 5 6 7 8 9 10

    Does not interfere — Completely interferes

13. Opening your mouth widely

    0 1 2 3 4 5 6 7 8 9 10

    Does not interfere — Completely interferes

14. Eating hard foods like apples

    0 1 2 3 4 5 6 7 8 9 10

    Does not interfere — Completely interferes

Circle the ONE number that describes your pain at its WORST in the last week.

0 1 2 3 4 5 6 7 8 9 10

No Pain — Pain as bad as you can imagine

Circle the ONE number that describes your pain at its LEAST in the last week.

0 1 2 3 4 5 6 7 8 9 10

No Pain — Pain as bad as you can imagine

Circle the ONE number that describes your pain at its AVERAGE in the last week.

0 1 2 3 4 5 6 7 8 9 10

No Pain — Pain as bad as you can imagine

Circle the ONE number that describes your pain RIGHT NOW.

0 1 2 3 4 5 6 7 8 9 10

No Pain — Pain as bad as you can imagine

Fig. 3. PFPS.

(see **Table 2**).[6,35] Although the recommendations are designed for clinical research trials, it is imperative to have a uniform format for measuring pain in the clinical practice setting.

Minimal Clinically Important Difference

An important step in selecting a standard scale is choosing a PRO that can detect a change in score that is clinically significant or meaningful. The change in score on the scale that is meaningful to the patient is known as the minimal clinically important difference (MCID). The MCID has been defined by Jaeschke and colleagues[38] as the "smallest difference in score in the domain of interest which patients perceive as beneficial and which would mandate, in the absence of troublesome side effects and excessive cost, a change in the patient's management."

Although it is important to have a tool that is both reliable and valid over time, it is equally as important for it to detect the MCID.[39] To determine the MCID, an external criterion is typically used as an objective assessment that can be compared with the change in score on the PRO.[5] The external criterion in the setting of pain can be a global assessment, such as the Patient Global Impression of Change. Global assessments are the superlative measure for obtaining the patient's perspective of the change in their clinical status.[40]

It is critical to determine the MCID because studies with statistically significant results may bear no clinical relevance. The contrary is also true: a clinically significant change for the patient may not be statistically significant.[41,42] Many clinicians may also think that they can intuitively sense a clinically significant change in their patients; however, clinicians may actually overestimate the benefits of treatment.[1,43] Therefore, it is essential to determine the MCID so that it is easier to decipher whether or not a patient has a meaningful change after their treatment. The MCID is also useful for health care professionals who are less acquainted with the scale, making it easier for them to interpret outcomes and decipher whether or not the patient has achieved the MCID.[38]

The MCID has been determined for some of the selected PROs evaluated in this article.

Visual Analog Scale

Reddy and colleagues[11,12] determined the MCID for the VAS in patients who had undergone RFL and MVD. The calculated MCIDs were 4.13-point to 8.2-point and 1.4-point to 8.87-point reductions in score, respectively.

It is significant that 2 of the 3 external criteria used by Reddy and colleagues to calculate the MCID did not have established psychometric properties; therefore, the MCID values may not be reliable or valid.

Numeric Rating Scale

In a study of 10 clinical trials of pregabalin in 5 chronic pain diseases (diabetic neuropathy, postherpetic neuralgia, chronic low back pain, fibromyalgia, and osteoarthritis), there was a consistent relationship between the NRS and the Patient Global Impression of Change.[44] In the same study, the MCID for the NRS was determined to be a 2-point reduction or a 30% reduction in score.[45] The MCID has also been determined in a study of TN patients. The results of the study found that the MCID for NRS–average pain intensity was a 2-point reduction or a 28% reduction in score.[46] The congruity of the results support the external validity of the MCID for the NRS because various chronic pain conditions have similar results.

Barrow Neurological Institute Pain Intensity Score

Reddy and colleagues determined the MCID for the BNI-PS in patients who had undergone RFL and MVD. The MCIDs were 1.03-point to 3.30-point and 0.95-point to 3.26-point reductions in score, respectively.

The validity and reliability of the BNI-PS scale have not been verified. Consequently, even though the MCID has been determined for the scale, the calculated values may not be reliable. In addition, Reddy and colleagues used the same external criteria used to calculate the MCID for the VAS; therefore, the same issues of reliability and validity of MCID values are present with this scale.

McGill Pain Questionnaire

The MCIDs for the 3 indices of the MPQ (pain rating index, total number of words selected, and PPI) have not been determined.

Penn Facial Pain Scale

After the psychometric properties of the scale were established, the MCID was determined for the 3 components of the PFPS. The MCID was a 3.7-point reduction or 75% reduction in score for general interference and a 2.3-point reduction or 62% reduction in score for facial interference. The MCID was a 6-point reduction or 57% reduction in score for NRS–worst pain intensity, and a 2-point reduction or 28% reduction in score for NRS–average pain intensity.[46]

SUMMARY AND RECOMMENDATIONS

There is no simple, universally accepted method to measure pain in patients with TN. The VAS and NRS are simple to understand and easy to administer but suffer perhaps from being too simple and 1-D. And although the MPQ is comprehensive, its reliance on vocabulary and descriptors may be challenging for some individuals. The BNI-PS has excellent face validity but lacks proper instrument design, and its psychometric properties have not been validated. Hence, the PFPS, which includes the Brief Pain Inventory, seems a solid option for measurement of pain in patients with TN.

Given the importance of multidimensional measurement of pain outcomes, it makes sense to combine outcome tools. The solution for this issue could be a single questionnaire that combines multiple PROs. Individually, each scale that was evaluated in this article either lacked components of Deyo's recommendations or only partially adhered to the IMMPACT recommendations. An optimal questionnaire could be created by combining scales that have established psychometric properties, calculated MCIDs, and compliance with Deyo's and IMMPACT recommendations.

Zakrzweska and colleagues[47] developed the first composite questionnaire that could be used to evaluate outcomes in the surgical TN population. The scale was developed after consulting with patients, neurosurgeons, statisticians, and sociologists and an extensive review of TN literature. The questionnaire was a combination of the Short Form (SF)-12, Hospital Anxiety and Depression Scale (HAD) score, BPI, and MPQ. The SF-12 has been adapted from the SF-36, which is a medical outcomes scale with a bodily pain section that has been used to measure pain.[48] The HAD has known sensitivity for changes in TN pain.[49,50] The questionnaire was distributed to patients of a single center. The researchers had a 92% response rate (n = 305) and the results were reproducible. The questionnaire was then modified to improve its validity. The new scale was called the Annual Trigeminal Neuralgia Survey. The revised survey applies to 5 of the 6 domains of the IMMPACT recommendations and is only lacking a global improvement or satisfaction rating. The revised questionnaire has yet to be studied; however, if the psychometric properties and MCID were determined for the scale, it could be an excellent option for evaluating outcomes in the TN population.

A more streamlined questionnaire could be developed by combining the PFPS, HAD, Patient Global Impression of Change, and an open-ended form for symptoms and disposition. The combination of scales and open-ended form applies to all 6 of the IMMPACT domains. This combination creates a comprehensive questionnaire that has minimal patient and administrative burden and could be easily dispersed to TN patients to assess their change in clinical status and outcomes.

Although there are many PROs that can be used for measuring TN pain and response to treatment, review of the available literature has proved that there is a lack of utilization of PROs and poor quality of reporting TN outcomes. To better assess patient outcomes and efficacy of treatments, it is essential that a standard questionnaire be developed and used universally in both the clinical and research setting. Researchers are encouraged to use the PFPS at to assess neurosurgical and medical outcomes in patients with TN.

ACKNOWLEDGMENTS

Sukhmeet K. Sandhu, BA, Department of Neurosurgery, University of Pennsylvania, Philadelphia, PA, contributed to the writing of this article.

REFERENCES

1. Turk DC, Rudy TE, Sorkin BA. Neglected topics in chronic pain treatment outcome studies: determination of success. Pain 1993;53:3–16. Available at: http://linkinghub.elsevier.com/retrieve/pii/030439599390049U.
2. Baron R, Binder A, Wasner G. Neuropathic pain: diagnosis, pathophysiological mechanisms, and treatment. Lancet Neurol 2010;9(8):807–19.
3. Farrar JT, Portenoy RK, Berlin JA, et al. Defining the clinically important difference in pain outcome measures. Pain 2000;88(3):287–94.
4. Turk DC, Melzack R. Handbook of pain assessment. 2nd edition. New York: The Guilford Press; 2001.
5. Copay AG, Subach BR, Glassman SD, et al. Understanding the minimum clinically important difference: a review of concepts and methods. Spine J 2007;7:541–6.
6. Dworkin RH, Turk DC, Wyrwich KW, et al. Interpreting the clinical importance of treatment outcomes in chronic pain clinical trials: IMMPACT recommendations. J Pain 2008;9:105–21.
7. Price DD, McGrath PA, Rafii A, et al. The validation of visual analogue scales as ratio scale measures for chronic and experimental pain. Pain 1983;17(1):45–56.
8. Price DD, Bush FM, Long S, et al. A comparison of pain measurement characteristics of mechanical visual analogue and simple numerical rating scales. Pain 1994;56(2):217–26.
9. Jorns TP, Johnston A, Zakrzewska JM. Pilot study to evaluate the efficacy and tolerability of levetiracetam (Keppra) in treatment of patients with trigeminal neuralgia. Eur J Neurol 2009;16(6):740–4.
10. Jawahar A, Wadhwa R, Berk C, et al. Assessment of pain control, quality of life, and predictors of success after gamma knife surgery for the treatment

of trigeminal neuralgia. Neurosurg Focus 2005; 18(5):E8.
11. Reddy VK, Parker SL, Lockney DT, et al. Percutaneous stereotactic radiofrequency lesioning for trigeminal neuralgia: determination of minimum clinically important difference in pain improvement for patient-reported outcomes. Neurosurgery 2014; 74:262–6.
12. Reddy VK, Parker SL, Patrawala SA, et al. Microvascular decompression for classic trigeminal neuralgia: determination of minimum clinically important difference in pain improvement for patient reported outcomes. Neurosurgery 2013;72(5):749–54.
13. Stevens SS. Psychophysics: introduction to its perceptual, neural, and social prospects. 1975. doi:10.2307/1421904.
14. de C Williams AC, Davies HT, Chadury Y. Simple pain rating scales hide complex idiosyncratic meanings. Pain 2000;85(3):457–63.
15. Jensen MP, Karoly P, Braver S. The measurement of clinical pain intensity: a comparison of six methods. Pain 1986;27(1):117–26.
16. Paice JA, Cohen FL. Validity of a verbally administered numeric rating scale to measure cancer pain intensity. Cancer Nurs 1997;20(2):88–93.
17. Jaeschke R, Singer J, Guyatt GH. A comparison of seven-point and visual analogue scales. Data from a randomized trial. Control Clin Trials 1990;11(1): 43–51.
18. Juniper EF, Guyatt GH, Willan A, et al. Determining a minimal important change in a disease-specific Quality of Life Questionnaire. J Clin Epidemiol 1994;47:81–7.
19. Rogers CL, Shetter AG, Fiedler JA, et al. Gamma knife radiosurgery for trigeminal neuralgia: the initial experience of The Barrow Neurological Institute. Int J Radiat Oncol Biol Phys 2000;47:1013–9.
20. Park SH, Hwang SK. Outcomes of gamma knife radiosurgery for trigeminal neuralgia after a minimum 3-year follow-up. J Clin Neurosci 2011;18(5):645–8.
21. McNatt SA, Yu C, Giannotta SL, et al. Gamma knife radiosurgery for trigeminal neuralgia. Neurosurgery 2005;56(6):1295–301.
22. Reading AE, Everitt BS, Sledmere CM. The McGill Pain Questionnaire: a replication of its construction. Br J Clin Psychol 1982;21:339–49.
23. Burchiel KJ, Anderson VC, Brown FD, et al. Prospective, multicenter study of spinal cord stimulation for relief of chronic back and extremity pain. Spine (Phila Pa 1976) 1996;21(23):2786–94. Available at: http://journals.lww.com/spinejournal/Abstract/1996/12010/Prospective,_Multicenter_Study_of_Spinal_Cord.15.aspxn.
24. Love A, Leboeuf C, Crisp TC. Chiropractic chronic low back pain sufferers and self-report assessment methods. Part I. A reliability study of the Visual Analogue Scale, the Pain Drawing and the McGill Pain Questionnaire. J Manipulative Physiol Ther 1989;12(2):21–5.
25. Melzack R, Terrence C, Fromm G, et al. Trigeminal neuralgia and atypical facial pain: use of the McGill Pain Questionnaire for discrimination and diagnosis. Pain 1986;27(3):297–302.
26. Zakrzewska JM. Diagnosis and differential diagnosis of trigeminal neuralgia. Clin J Pain 2002;18(1):14–21.
27. Szapiro J, Sindou M, Szapiro J. Prognostic factors in microvascular decompression for trigeminal neuralgia. Neurosurgery 1985;17(6):920–9.
28. Zakrzewska JM, Lopez BC. Quality of reporting in evaluations of surgical treatment of trigeminal neuralgia: recommendations for future reports. Neurosurgery 2003;53:110–20 [discussion: 120–2].
29. Cleeland CS, Ryan KM. Pain assessment: global use of the Brief Pain Inventory. Ann Acad Med Singapore 1994;23:129–38.
30. Keller S, Bann CM, Dodd SL, et al. Validity of the brief pain inventory for use in documenting the outcomes of patients with noncancer pain. Clin J Pain 2004;20:309–18.
31. Tan G, Jensen MP, Thornby JI, et al. Validation of the brief pain inventory for chronic nonmalignant pain. J Pain 2004;5(2):133–7.
32. Engel JM, Schwartz L, Jensen MP, et al. Pain in cerebral palsy: the relation of coping strategies to adjustment. Pain 2000;88(3):225–30.
33. Chen H, Lee J. The measurement of pain in patients with trigeminal neuralgia. Clin Neurosurg 2010;57: 129–33.
34. Lee JYK, Chen HI, Urban C, et al. Development of and psychometric testing for the Brief Pain Inventory-Facial in patients with facial pain syndromes. J Neurosurg 2010;113:516–23.
35. Dworkin R, Farrar J. Research design issues in pain clinical trials. Neurology 2005;65(12) Suppl 4: S1–2. Available at: http://www.neurology.org/content/65/12_suppl_4/S1.short.
36. Deyo RA. Measuring functional outcomes in therapeutic trials for chronic disease. Control Clin Trials 1984;5(3):223–40.
37. Deyo RA, Centor RM. Assessing the responsiveness of functional scales to clinical change: an analogy to diagnostic test performance. J Chronic Dis 1986;39: 897–906.
38. Jaeschke R, Singer J, Guyatt GH. Measurement of health status. Ascertaining the minimal clinically important difference. Control Clin Trials 1989;10(4):407–15.
39. Guyatt G, Walter S, Norman G. Measuring change over time: assessing the usefulness of evaluative instruments. J Chronic Dis 1987;40(2):171–8.
40. Crosby RD, Kolotkin RL, Williams GR. Defining clinically meaningful change in health-related quality of life. J Clin Epidemiol 2003;56:395–407.
41. Bolton JE. Sensitivity and specificity of outcome measures in patients with neck pain: detecting

clinically significant improvement. Spine (Phila Pa 1976) 2004;29:2410–7 [discussion: 2418].

42. Jacobson NS, Follette WC, Revenstorf D. Psychotherapy outcome research: methods for reporting variability and evaluating clinical significance. Behav Ther 1984;15(4):336–52.

43. Daniel M. Therapists' and chronic pain patients' perceptions of treatment outcome. J Nerv Ment Dis 1983;171(12):729–33. Available at: http://ovidsp.ovid.com/ovidweb.cgi?T=JS&CSC=Y&NEWS=N&PAGE=fulltext&D=psyc2&AN=1984-10005 001n http://nhs5195535.resolver.library.nhs.uk/?sid=OVID:psycdb&id=pmid:&id=doi:10.1097/00005053-198312000-00004&issn=0022-3018&isbn=&volume=171&issue=12&spage=729&pa.

44. Farrar JT, Pritchett YL, Robinson M, et al. The clinical importance of changes in the 0 to 10 numeric rating scale for worst, least, and average pain intensity: analyses of data from clinical trials of duloxetine in pain disorders. J Pain 2010;11(2):109–18.

45. Farrar JT, Young JP, LaMoreaux L, et al. Clinical importance of changes in chronic pain intensity measured on an 11-point numerical pain rating scale. Pain 2001;94(2):149–58.

46. Sandhu SK, Halpern CH, Vakhshori V, et al. Brief Pain Inventory–Facial minimum clinically important difference. J Neurosurg 2015;122(1):180–90.

47. Zakrzewska JM, Lopez BC, Kim SE, et al. Patient satisfaction after surgery for trigeminal neuralgia–development of a questionnaire. Acta Neurochir (Wien) 2005;147(9):925–32.

48. Hawker GA, Mian S, Kendzerska T, et al. Measures of adult pain: Visual Analog Scale for Pain (VAS Pain), Numeric Rating Scale for Pain (NRS Pain), McGill Pain Questionnaire (MPQ), Short-Form McGill Pain Questionnaire (SF-MPQ), Chronic Pain Grade Scale (CPGS), Short Form-36 Bodily Pain Scale (SF-36 BPS), and Measure of Intermittent and Constant Osteoarthritis Pain (ICOAP). Arthritis Care Res 2011;63(Suppl 11):S240–52.

49. Zakrzewska JM, Thomas DG. Patient's assessment of outcome after three surgical procedures for the management of trigeminal neuralgia. Acta Neurochir (Wien) 1993;122(3–4):225–30.

50. Zakrzewska JM, Jassim S, Bulman JS. A prospective, longitudinal study on patients with trigeminal neuralgia who underwent radiofrequency thermocoagulation of the Gasserian ganglion. Pain 1999;79(1):51–8.

Management of Skull Base Tumor–Associated Facial Pain

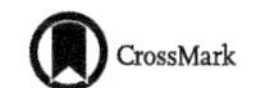

Gaddum Duemani Reddy, MD, PhD[a], Kathryn Wagner, MD[a], Jack Phan, MD, PhD[b], Franco DeMonte, MD[a], Shaan M. Raza, MD[a,*]

KEYWORDS

• Trigeminal neuralgia • Cancer pain • Surgical treatment • Medical treatment • Radiation therapy

KEY POINTS

- Intracranial tumors and head and neck tumors can be frequently associated with facial pain through a variety of mechanisms.
- Effective medical treatment of cancer-associated facial pain is achieved through treatment of the underlying tumor as well as treatment of associated symptoms.
- Radiosurgery treatment can be both a source and a cure for facial pain associated with cancer.
- Surgery is often the most effective treatment of cancer-associated pain and includes both tumor resection as well as destructive procedures.

INTRODUCTION

Tumor-associated facial pain is a complex diagnosis that does not lend itself to easy classification. Modern classifications are moving away from terms such as *typical* and *atypical* facial pain in favor of those that convey a deeper understanding of the underlying etiology.[1] Attempting to categorize the facial pain that accompanies tumors is complicated, however, by the myriad ways in which tumors can cause this pain. These causes include perineural tumor invasion, mucosal irritation, infection/inflammation, soft tissue invasion, and necrosis.[2,3] Further complicating the picture are the side effects of standard cancer treatments, specifically chemotherapy, radiation, and surgery, which can either alleviate facial pain or cause/worsen it. To better characterize this complex and unique type of facial pain, the authors divide the tumors that cause facial pain into 3 types based on the anatomy and describe the symptoms associated with these categories. The authors then discuss the effectiveness and drawbacks of various treatment modalities, including medication/chemotherapy, radiosurgery, and surgery.

CATEGORIES OF SKULL BASE TUMORS ASSOCIATED WITH FACIAL PAIN

One of the simplest methods of classifying the variety of tumors associated with facial pain is by anatomic location along the trigeminal system. Using this paradigm, the most common lesions are posterior cranial fossa tumors (trigeminal root), middle cranial fossa tumors (gasserian ganglion and trigeminal divisions), and head and neck tumors (trigeminal divisions and distal branches). Additionally, distal tumors can result in trigeminal neuralgia; these will also be briefly discussed later.

Disclosure Statement: The authors have nothing to disclose.
[a] Department of Neurosurgery, The University of Texas M.D. Anderson Cancer Center, 1515 Holcombe Boulevard, Houston, TX 77030, USA; [b] Department of Radiation Oncology, The University of Texas M.D. Anderson Cancer Center, 1515 Holcombe Boulevard, Houston, TX 77030, USA
* Corresponding author.
E-mail address: SMRaza@mdanderson.org

Neurosurg Clin N Am 27 (2016) 337–344
http://dx.doi.org/10.1016/j.nec.2016.02.009
1042-3680/16/$ – see front matter

Each of these categories can present with facial or trigeminal pain through a variety of mechanisms, and the incidence at each anatomic location can be estimated from large published case series (**Table 1**).

Posterior and Middle Cranial Fossa Tumors

Classically, intracranial tumors are associated with a "brain tumor headache," which has been defined by the International Headache Society as progressive, worse in the morning, and aggravated by Valsalvalike maneuvers.[4] Intracranial mass lesions often compress and obstruct cerebral spinal fluid pathways, leading to the aforementioned symptoms of elevated intracranial pressure. However, although the correlation between brain tumors and headaches is well established, with incidences ranging upwards of 70%[5] for both metastatic and primary tumors, this classic "brain tumor headache" has been shown in recent studies to happen infrequently.[6]

Instead, skull base tumors can present with a variety of pain syndromes, including facial pain that is often diagnosed as trigeminal neuralgia. The constellation of symptoms seen in this cohort can not only be that of typical trigeminal neuralgia (ie, sharp lancinating pain with clear triggers) but also associated with a neuropathy (ie, decreased sensation in any one of the trigeminal divisions or masseter dysfunction). This has been well described in the literature in various case reports, particularly for tumors of the cerebellopontine angle.[7,8] Larger studies have also been done to confirm this, but have shown variable rates of incidence. For example, in a retrospective series from the Mayfield clinic, only 0.8% of 2000 patients with facial pain were found to have an intracranial tumor,[9] with peripherally located tumors causing atypical facial pain associated with a sensory loss and middle/posterior fossa tumors causing trigeminal neuralgia symptoms. On the other hand, in a 15-year retrospective review of more than 5000 patients evaluated for facial pain at the Mayo Clinic, more than 2900 patients were diagnosed with trigeminal neuralgia and nearly 6% were found to have causal intracranial masses, most commonly in the posterior fossa.[10] Examples of tumors in the posterior and middle cranial fossa that can present with trigeminal neuralgia are shown in **Table 2**.

Table 1
Tumors associated with facial pain: symptoms and incidences

	Symptoms	Incidence
Intracranial tumors	Headache, TN, TAC	70%
Head and neck tumors	Orofacial pain, TN	80%
Distal tumors	Neuropathies	Rare

Abbreviations: TAC, trigeminal autonomic cephalalgia; TN, trigeminal neuralgia.

With tumors of the posterior fossa (ie, petroclival meningiomas, vestibular schwannomas) and middle fossa (ie, trigeminal schwannoma) (**Fig. 1**), direct mechanical compression of the trigeminal root is thought to be the primary pain generator. A similar mechanism can also be seen with middle fossa tumors (see **Fig. 1**). Of note, with prolongation of time without treatment, this prolonged mechanical compression is thought to result in breakdown in Schwann cells and axonal degeneration. On the other hand, histologic studies of cavernous meningiomas have demonstrated tumor invasion of the perineural layer of involved cranial nerves. This phenomenon can be independent of histologic grade and likely represents another mechanism of tumor: associated trigeminal neuralgia beyond the standard mechanical compression seen with benign tumors of the middle and posterior cranial fossa.

More recent studies have also shown an association between brain tumors and trigeminal autonomic cephalalgias (TACs). These TACs are recently described entities by the International Headache Society that resemble trigeminal neuralgia but encompass a unilateral facial pain syndrome with an associated ipsilateral autonomic dysfunction. Although most often associated with pituitary tumors,[11–13] TACs have also been reported in other tumors that invade the cavernous sinus.[14–16]

Head and Neck Tumors

Head and neck malignancies can also present with facial pain. The rich network of distal trigeminal nerve branches along the skin and within the subcranial structures (ie, nasal cavity, paranasal sinuses, pterygopalatine fossa, infratemporal fossa) exposes them to the risk of perineural invasion (PNI) with neurotrophic cancers (**Table 3**). PNI represents a mode of cancer spread whereby tumor cells invade the perineural space and spread along those nerves to distant locations. Clinical PNI refers to a clinical deficit on presentation as a result of tumor spread involved in a large named nerve (ie, infraorbital nerve, buccal nerve). Regardless, the presence of clinical or radiographic PNI must be accounted for during any oncologic treatment. For nonmelanoma cutaneous malignancies, the rates of PNI can vary; but up to 14% of

Table 2
Examples of intracranial skull base tumors associated with trigeminal neuralgia (organized by anatomic division of the trigeminal nerve)

Trigeminal Root	Gasserian Ganglion	Trigeminal Divisions
Petroclival meningioma	Trigeminal schwannoma	Trigeminal schwannoma
Vestibular schwannoma	Petroclival meningioma with Meckel cave extension	Meningioma
Trigeminal schwannoma	Chondrosarcoma	Head and neck malignancy with perineural invasion
Jugular foramen schwannoma	Chordoma	
Epidermoid	Cholesterol granuloma	
	Head and neck malignancy with perineural invasion	

squamous cell carcinomas and 10% of basal cell carcinomas can have evidence of clinical or radiographic perineural involvement.[17] Additionally, advanced malignancies of the paranasal sinuses, such as adenoid cystic carcinoma, are characterized by profound neurotrophic behavior.[18] Involvement of V2 (and its branches) can be seen with anatomic involvement of the maxillary sinus and pterygopalatine fossa, whereas invasion of V3 and its trunks/branches is typically of concern with tumor involvement of the oropharynx/nasopharynx, the infratemporal fossa, the parotid gland, and the mandible (**Fig. 2**). Histologically, evidence of the PNI is seen; areas of axonal injury and segmental nerve infarction can also be demonstrated, indicating the permanent injury that can result in untreatable pain. Outside of PNI, deep tumors of the nasopharynx and oropharynx can cause trigeminal neuralgia by direct nerve compression.[19] Systemic tumors, including lymphoma[20,21] and myeloma,[22,23] can cause localized pain in the facial region when they invade bone and soft tissue. Although neuropathy from direct infiltration of the nerves by leukemic cells is rare, it too has also been reported and is termed *neuroleukemiosis*.[24]

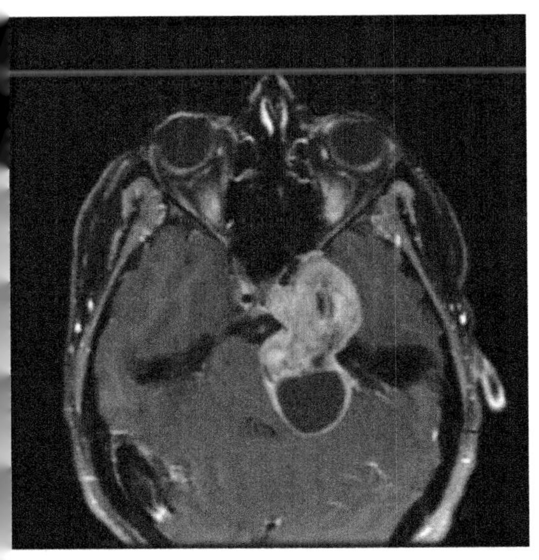

Fig. 1. This image is of a patient presenting with left-sided trigeminal neuralgia involving the V1, V2, and V3 distribution along with papilledema from obstructive hydrocephalus. Imaging shown demonstrates a large left-sided trigeminal schwannoma with disease in the Meckel cave in addition to the posterior fossa. Patient was treated surgically via an orbitozygomatic craniotomy with an anterior petrosectomy. (*Courtesy of* Department of Neurosurgery, The University of Texas M.D. Anderson Cancer Center, Houston, TX.)

In cases of clinical PNI, patients typically present with atypical forms of trigeminal neuralgia. The primary complaint is of formication and/or burning pain that initially involves distal branches (ie, greater palatine nerve with nasopharyngeal lesions, buccal nerve with oropharyngeal lesions) and then spread with time and without treatment to more proximal trunks (ie, anterolateral trunk for V3) and divisions of the trigeminal system (**Fig. 3**). Clinical involvement of all 3 divisions raises concern for involvement of the gasserian ganglion. A careful history and examination is important to not only delineate the extent of cranial nerve involvement but also to ensure that these patients are not treated as having classic trigeminal neuralgia. A radiographic evaluation with a high-resolution MRI scan with fat saturation helps characterize the extent of nerve involvement. Findings of contrast enhancement and/or enlargement of the nerve with obliteration of fat planes at the foramina suggest PNI. Additionally, involvement of the motor nerves (ie, posterolateral trunk of V3) can present with denervation changes of the end musculature consisting of abnormal contrast enhancement and T2 hyperintensity of the muscles.

Although not the focus of this article, it is imperative to highlight the prognostic impact of PNI.

Table 3
Examples of head and neck malignancies associated with perineural invasion classified by trigeminal division and subcranial compartment

Trigeminal Division	Subcranial Compartment	Histologic Diagnosis
V1 division	Orbit	Squamous cell carcinoma Neurotropic melanoma Adenoid cystic carcinoma (lacrimal gland)
V2 division	Pterygopalatine fossa Nasopharynx/palate Maxillary sinus	Nasopharyngeal carcinoma Squamous cell Adenoid cystic carcinoma Sinonasal undifferentiated carcinoma
V3 division	Infratemporal fossa Oropharynx	High-grade sarcoma Squamous cell carcinoma of the parotid gland Oropharyngeal carcinoma Adenoid cystic carcinoma

Note that compartments listed exclude cutaneous regions supplied by each trigeminal division.

Clinical PNI with radiographic evidence is associated with reduced 5-year progression-free survival for cutaneous malignancies. Similar findings are found for sinonasal malignancies. However, the negative impact of PNI can be partially negated by carefully designed surgical approaches that yield negative margins or radiation fields to provide coverage distally along the involved nerve.[17,25]

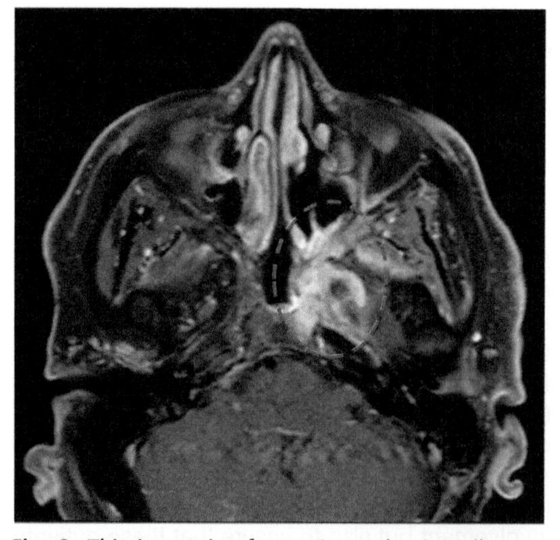

Fig. 2. This image is of a patient who initially presented with left V2 and V3 neuropathy in addition to formication. Patient initially underwent a microvascular decompression at an outside institution. After the development of ipsilateral facial nerve weakness, the patient presented to the authors' institution. Imaging shown (MRI axial T1-weighted with contrast) demonstrated abnormal tissue within the pterygopalatine fossa and infratemporal fossa (*dashed red circle*) with enhancement along the infraorbital nerve in addition to the greater superficial petrosal nerve. Endoscopic transpterygoid biopsy confirmed the diagnosis of invasive squamous cell carcinoma with PNI. Patient was treated with chemoradiation therapy. (*Courtesy of* Department of Neurosurgery, The University of Texas M.D. Anderson Cancer Center, Houston, TX.)

Distal Tumors

Among the rarest tumors to cause facial pain are cancers that do not directly involve the intracranial cavity or the head/neck. However, facial pain has been reported as consequence of several types of tumors, including lung [26,27] and pancreatic cancers[28] that do not directly metastasize to the skull or face. The cause of this pain has been suggested to arise from compression of the vagus nerve, leading to facial pain secondary to convergence of these fibers with fibers from the trigeminal tract. Alternatively, distal tumors, particularly small cell lung cancer or systemic tumors, can induce a paraneoplastic syndrome, which has also been associated with sensory neuropathy presenting as facial pain.[29]

TREATMENT OF TUMOR-ASSOCIATED FACIAL PAIN

Treatment of the facial pain symptoms that accompany tumors is not simple. Largely this is because modalities designed to treat the underlying tumor, including chemotherapy, radiosurgery, and surgical resection, have been associated with both eliminating facial pain and initiating facial pain in patients who previously had none. Additionally, the mechanism of pain (ie, PNI) can result in situations whereby the primary treatment will not treat the associated pain syndrome. As a result, the expectations for the management of facial pain have to be separated from the primary

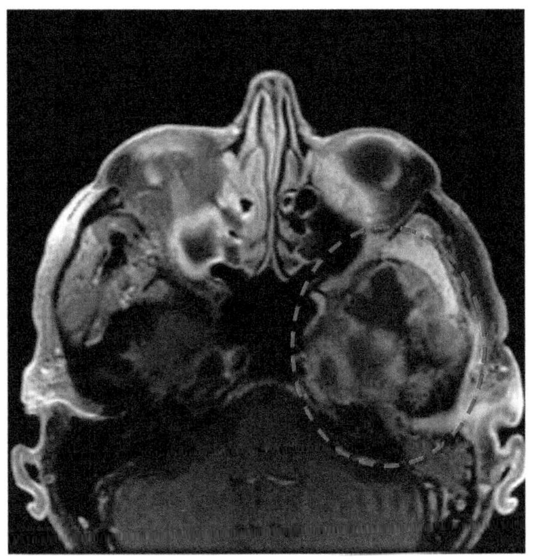

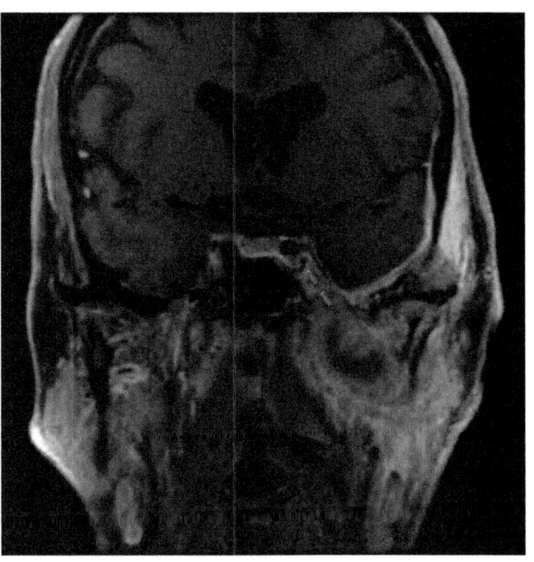

Fig. 3. This image is of a patient who was initially treated by Mohs and radiation therapy for squamous cell carcinoma of the preauricular skin. Three years after treatment, the patient developed facial nerve weakness with pain in the left V2/V3 distribution in addition to trismus. Imaging on the left (MRI axial T1 weighted with contrast) demonstrates disease within the infratemporal fossa in addition to the middle cranial fossa (*dashed red circle*). Coronal imaging on the right demonstrates PNI along V3 through foramen ovale into the Meckel's cave (*dashed red line*). Patient was treated with induction chemotherapy followed by a subtemporal-infratemporal fossa resection and adjuvant radiation therapy. (*Courtesy of* Department of Neurosurgery, The University of Texas M.D. Anderson Cancer Center, Houston, TX.)

oncological treatment, particularly for skull base malignancies. To simplify this, the authors divide treatments into 3 categories: medical, radiosurgical, and surgical. Each category has a reported range of effectiveness in treating the facial pain that often accompanies cancer (see **Table 2**). Similarly, each category has an associated incidence of causing trigeminal pain, which can also be estimated from larger case studies.

Medical

Medical therapy for intracranial tumor-associated facial pain and headaches can further be subdivided into 2 categorizes: symptomatic therapy and curative therapy.

Symptomatic therapy

Symptomatic therapy for facial pain related to cancer proceeds along 2 separate paths. The first uses the World Health Organization's (WHO) ladder, in which non-narcotic pain medications, including nonsteroidal antiinflammatory drugs, are first implemented, followed by mild narcotics, such as hydrocodone and oxycodone, and finally heavier narcotics, such as morphine and hydromorphone. Using this protocol, a large percentage of all cancer pain can be controlled.[30] The second path, which is also included as adjuvant therapy in the WHO's system, uses medications that are typically used for neuropathic pain or trigeminal neuralgia, including gabapentin[31] and carbamazepine. It also includes medications for relieving treatment-induced oral mucositis. Indeed, topical agents, including benzydamine[32] and doxepin,[33] have been shown to improve pain when applied to the mucosal membranes affected by mucositis from either radiation or chemotherapy treatments.

Curative therapy

Curative therapy relates to the use of medications designed to treat the underlying tumor. Classically, this would describe chemotherapy; but there is sparse information in the literature regarding the improvement in facial pain with systemic chemotherapy. Instead, the most described situation in the literature is the use of dopamine agonists in patients with prolactinomas. The results in this situation, however, have been inconsistent. Indeed, at least 3 case reports have shown significant improvement in TAC symptoms after the initiation of cabergoline.[16,34,35] On the other hand, in the study by Levy and colleagues[11] involving 23 patients treated with cabergoline for prolactinomas, symptomatic improvement was seen in only 9 patients, whereas 11 had no improvement and 3 reported worsening symptoms. Similarly, the use of bromocriptine was also more often associated with either no significant changes in the headache symptoms or worsening of these symptoms. This larger study recapitulated the results found in earlier case reports by the same group showing exacerbation of TAC symptoms in patients treated with dopamine agonists.[36,37] Less well described in the literature has been the effectiveness of symptomatic improvement with use of octreotide for the treatment of acromegaly. In the study by Levy and colleagues, whereby 22 patients with acromegaly were treated with either octreotide or lanreotide, a similar somatostatin analogue, 12 patients reported improvement in symptoms.[11]

Radiosurgery

Over the past 2 decades, radiosurgery has emerged as a potential treatment option for trigeminal pain, including pain secondary to tumor. Pollack and colleagues[38] reported their results on 24 patients treated with radiosurgery for tumors causing symptoms of facial pain. In their series, 50% reported resolution of symptoms and another 46% reported reduction in symptoms.[38] Similarly, in a series describing the effect of Gamma Knife (Elektra Instruments, Stockholm, Sweden) radiosurgery on facial pain secondary to intracranial meningiomas and schwannomas, Huang and colleagues[39] reported that approximately 60% had pain relief without medication after one round of Gamma Knife radiosurgery. After a repeat session, however, nearly 75% had a significant improvement in their facial pain.

It is important to note 2 confounding factors in these results. The first is that the durability of the improvement is debatable. Indeed, in a long-term study by Chang and colleagues,[40] although 85% of patient with tumor-associated facial pain from primarily cerebellopontine angle tumors had initial improvement, approximately half had recurrence. This finding is recapitulated in work done by Tanaka and colleagues,[41] who showed that, although approximately 60% of patients with skull base tumors who underwent radiosurgery had complete resolution of pain, only 25% had durable relief at the last follow-up. The second is that radiosurgery is becoming a more common primary treatment of brain tumors. Although radiosurgery often improves isolated trigeminal neuralgia, it has also been noted that trigeminal neuralgia can develop after radiosurgery treatment, particularly for tumors of the cerebellopontine or petroclival tumors.[42]

In unpublished work done at the MD Anderson Cancer Center (Phan J, DeMonte F, unpublished data, 2015), 20 patients with previously treated and irradiated malignant tumors of the head and neck were treated with radiosurgery for palliation of trigeminal facial pain. Sixteen patients were assessed for symptom palliation with a median follow-up of 6.2 months (range 3.0–19.9 months). Fifteen patients received a single fraction with a median dose of 16 Gy (range 10–20 Gy) prescribed to the 50% isodose line (range 43%–55%). One patient was treated with 24 Gy in 3 fractions prescribed to 50%. At 3 months after radiosurgery, self-reported pain scores decreased from 4.92 ± 3.97 to 1.39 ± 2.17 ($P<.01$) and the frequency of analgesic used was significantly decreased. At 6 months, 6 of 10 patients were pain free and 4 were off all analgesics.

Surgical

Surgical therapy, when feasible, has been shown to result in the highest rate of symptomatic improvement for benign skull base tumors. Unfortunately, such findings have not been demonstrated in the management of head and neck or skull base malignancies with trigeminal invasion. Surgical therapy can be divided into 2 subcategories: resection and destructive procedures.

Surgical resection

In the Levy and colleagues[11] study described earlier, nearly half of all patients who underwent surgical resection for their pituitary tumors reported postoperative improvement in pain symptoms. Similar results were found in case reports[13] as well as in another large series of patients who underwent endonasal surgical resection of skull base tumors. In this series of primarily pituitary tumors, nearly half of patients reported complete resolution in preoperative headachelike symptoms and an additional 35% reported some improvement.[43] Outside of pituitary-associated tumors, TAC-associated symptoms have also been showed to completely resolve after resection of tumors occurring along the tentorium.[44,45] In addition, it has been shown that trigeminal neuralgia in patients with trigeminal schwannomas is significantly reduced in most patients after surgical resection. Indeed, in the large series by Chen and colleagues[46] of 55 patients with trigeminal schwannomas, in which 11 presented with facial pain, 100% were successfully improved after surgical resection. Similarly, Wanibuchi and colleagues[47] report that, in their series of 105 patients with trigeminal schwannomas, 22 out of 24 patients reported symptomatic improvement in facial pain after surgical resection.

These results, however, are mitigated by the fact that, similar to Gamma Knife surgery, postoperative pain is not uncommon following surgery and can persist, particularly after posterior fossa surgery.[48] This finding is particularly true for skull base surgery; in their series of 231 patients with skull base meningiomas who underwent surgery, Westerlund and colleagues[49] reported a wide range of trigeminal-associated complications, including a 16% rate of new trigeminal pain.

Destructive procedures

In patients for whom surgical resection is not a possibility, or in whom it has not provided surgical relief, destructive procedures, including rhizotomy[50,51] and cryoablation,[52] have been reported in the literature with success. Of note, although destructive procedures for primary trigeminal neuralgia have been extensively reported,[53] their use in cancer-related pain is much less well documented.

SUMMARY

In conclusion, tumor-associated facial pain characterizes a broad range of pathologic conditions and can be caused by a variety of mechanisms. However, anatomically these tumors can be divided into intracranial tumors, head and neck tumors, and distal tumors. For each of these categories, treatment strategies include symptomatic or curative treatment with medications, radiosurgery, and surgery. All of these methods have varying degrees of success in treating facial pain, and the approach to each patient must be individualized to achieve the best results.

ACKNOWLEDGMENTS

Patrick J. Hunt, BS, Department of Neurosurgery, The University of Texas M.D. Anderson Cancer Center, Houston, TX contributed to the writing of this article.

REFERENCES

1. Burchiel KJ. A new classification for facial pain. Neurosurgery 2003;53:1164–6 [discussion: 1166–67].
2. Romero-Reyes M, Teruel A, Ye Y. Cancer and referred facial pain. Curr Pain Headache Rep 2015;19:37.
3. Epstein JB, Elad S, Eliav E, et al. Orofacial pain in cancer: part II–clinical perspectives and management. J Dent Res 2007;86:506–18.
4. Headache Classification Committee of the International Headache Society (IHS). The international classification of headache disorders, 3rd edition (beta version). Cephalalgia Int J Headache 2013;33:629–808.
5. Kirby S, Purdy RA. Headache and brain tumors. Curr Neurol Neurosci Rep 2007;7:110–6.
6. Nelson S, Taylor LP. Headaches in brain tumor patients: primary or secondary? Headache 2014;54:776–85.
7. Mehrkhodavandi N, Green D, Amato R. Toothache caused by trigeminal neuralgia secondary to vestibular schwannoma: a case report. J Endod 2014;40:1691–4.
8. Matsuka Y, Fort ET, Merrill RL. Trigeminal neuralgia due to an acoustic neuroma in the cerebellopontine angle. J Orofac Pain 2000;14:147–51.
9. Bullitt E, Tew JM, Boyd J. Intracranial tumors in patients with facial pain. J Neurosurg 1986;64:865–71.
10. Cheng TM, Cascino TL, Onofrio BM. Comprehensive study of diagnosis and treatment of trigeminal neuralgia secondary to tumors. Neurology 1993;43:2298–302.
11. Levy MJ, Matharu MS, Meeran K, et al. The clinical characteristics of headache in patients with pituitary tumours. Brain J Neurol 2005;128:1921–30.
12. Zidverc-Trajkovic J, Vujovic S, Sundic A, et al. Bilateral SUNCT-like headache in a patient with prolactinoma responsive to lamotrigine. J Headache Pain 2009;10:469–72.
13. Leone M, Curone M, Mea E, et al. Cluster-tic syndrome resolved by removal of pituitary adenoma: the first case. Cephalalgia Int J Headache 2004;24:1088–9.
14. Trucco M, Mainardi F, Maggioni F, et al. Chronic paroxysmal hemicrania, hemicrania continua and SUNCT syndrome in association with other pathologies: a review. Cephalalgia Int J Headache 2004;24:173–84.
15. Kaphan E, Eusebio A, Donnet A, et al. Short-lasting, unilateral, neuralgiform headache attacks with conjunctival injection and tearing (SUNCT syndrome) and tumour of the cavernous sinus. Cephalalgia Int J Headache 2003;23:395–7.
16. Sarov M, Valade D, Jublanc C, et al. Chronic paroxysmal hemicrania in a patient with a macroprolactinoma. Cephalalgia Int J Headache 2006;26:738–41.
17. Raza SM, Ramakrishna R, Weber RS, et al. Nonmelanoma cutaneous cancers involving the skull base: outcomes of aggressive multimodal management. J Neurosurg 2015;123:781–8.
18. Ramakrishna R, Raza SM, Kupferman M, et al. Adenoid cystic carcinoma of the skull base: results with an aggressive multidisciplinary approach. J Neurosurg 2016;124(1):115–21.
19. Clark GT, Ram S. Orofacial pain and neurosensory disorders and dysfunction in cancer patients. Dent Clin North Am 2008;52:183–202, ix–x.
20. Parihar S, Garg RK, Narain P. Primary extra-nodal non-Hodgkin's lymphoma of gingiva: a diagnostic dilemma. J Oral Maxillofac Pathol 2013;17:320.
21. Webber B, Webber M, Keinan D. Extranodal large B cell lymphoma of the anterior maxilla. Case report and review of literature. N Y State Dent J 2015;81:34–8.

22. Oranger A, Carbone C, Izzo M, et al. Cellular mechanisms of multiple myeloma bone disease. Clin Dev Immunol 2013;2013:289458.
23. Troeltzsch M, Oduncu F, Mayr D, et al. Root resorption caused by jaw infiltration of multiple myeloma: report of a case and literature review. J Endod 2014;40:1260–4.
24. Reddy CG, Mauermann ML, Solomon BM, et al. Neuroleukemiosis: an unusual cause of peripheral neuropathy. Leuk Lymphoma 2012;53:2405–11.
25. DeMonte F, Hanna E. Transmaxillary exploration of the intracranial portion of the maxillary nerve in malignant perineural disease. Technical note. J Neurosurg 2007;107:672–7.
26. Sarlani E, Schwartz AH, Greenspan JD, et al. Facial pain as first manifestation of lung cancer: a case of lung cancer-related cluster headache and a review of the literature. J Orofac Pain 2003;17:262–7.
27. Capobianco DJ. Facial pain as a symptom of nonmetastatic lung cancer. Headache 1995;35:581–5.
28. Dach F, Oliveira FA, dos Santos AC, et al. Trigeminal neuralgia as the sole symptom of pancreatic cancer. Headache 2013;53:165–7.
29. Demarquay G, Didelot A, Rogemond V, et al. Facial pain as first manifestation of anti-Hu paraneoplastic syndrome. J Headache Pain 2010;11:355–7.
30. Jadad AR, Browman GP. The WHO analgesic ladder for cancer pain management. Stepping up the quality of its evaluation. JAMA 1995;274:1870–3.
31. Bar Ad V. Gabapentin for the treatment of cancer-related pain syndromes. Rev Recent Clin Trials 2010;5:174–8.
32. Epstein JB, Silverman S Jr, Paggiarino DA, et al. Benzydamine HCl for prophylaxis of radiation-induced oral mucositis: results from a multicenter, randomized, double-blind, placebo-controlled clinical trial. Cancer 2001;92:875–85.
33. Leenstra JL, Miller RC, Qin R, et al. Doxepin rinse versus placebo in the treatment of acute oral mucositis pain in patients receiving head and neck radiotherapy with or without chemotherapy: a phase III, randomized, double-blind trial (NCCTG-N09C6 [Alliance]). J Clin Oncol 2014;32:1571–7.
34. Negoro K, Kawai M, Tada Y, et al. A case of postprandial cluster-like headache with prolactinoma: dramatic response to cabergoline. Headache 2005;45:604–6.
35. Porta-Etessam J, Ramos-Carrasco A, Berbel-García A, et al. Clusterlike headache as first manifestation of a prolactinoma. Headache 2001;41:723–5.
36. Levy MJ, Matharu MS, Goadsby PJ. Prolactinomas, dopamine agonists and headache: two case reports. Eur J Neurol 2003;10:169–73.
37. Massiou H, Launay JM, Levy C, et al. SUNCT syndrome in two patients with prolactinomas and bromocriptine-induced attacks. Neurology 2002;58:1698–9.
38. Pollock BE, Iuliano BA, Foote RL, et al. Stereotactic radiosurgery for tumor-related trigeminal pain. Neurosurgery 2000;46:576–82 [discussion: 582–83].
39. Huang C-F, Tu H-T, Liu W-S, et al. Gamma Knife surgery for trigeminal pain caused by benign brain tumors. J Neurosurg 2008;109(Suppl):154–9.
40. Chang JW, Kim SH, Huh R, et al. The effects of stereotactic radiosurgery on secondary facial pain. Stereotact Funct Neurosurg 1999;72(Suppl 1):29–37.
41. Tanaka S, Pollock BE, Stafford SL, et al. Stereotactic radiosurgery for trigeminal pain secondary to benign skull base tumors. World Neurosurg 2013;80:371–7.
42. Gerganov VM, Giordano M, Elolf E, et al. Operative management of patients with radiosurgery-related trigeminal neuralgia: analysis of the surgical morbidity and pain outcome. Clin Neurol Neurosurg 2014;122:23–8.
43. Dusick JR, Esposito F, Mattozo CA, et al. Endonasal transsphenoidal surgery: the patient's perspective-survey results from 259 patients. Surg Neurol 2006;65:332–41 [discussion: 341–42].
44. Taub E, Argoff CE, Winterkorn JM, et al. Resolution of chronic cluster headache after resection of a tentorial meningioma: case report. Neurosurgery 1995;37:319–21 [discussion: 321–22].
45. Bigal ME, Rapoport AM, Camel M. Cluster headache as a manifestation of intracranial inflammatory myofibroblastic tumour: a case report with pathophysiological considerations. Cephalalgia Int J Headache 2003;23:124–8.
46. Chen LF, Yang Y, Yu XG, et al. Operative management of trigeminal neuromas: an analysis of a surgical experience with 55 cases. Acta Neurochir (Wien) 2014;156:1105–14.
47. Wanibuchi M, Fukushima T, Zomordi AR, et al. Trigeminal schwannomas: skull base approaches and operative results in 105 patients. Neurosurgery 2012;70:132–43 [discussion: 143–44].
48. De Gray LC, Matta BF. Acute and chronic pain following craniotomy: a review. Anaesthesia 2005;60:693–704.
49. Westerlund U, Linderoth B, Mathiesen T. Trigeminal complications arising after surgery of cranial base meningiomas. Neurosurg Rev 2012;35:203–9 [discussion: 209–10].
50. Frank F, Tognetti F, Gaist G, et al. Percutaneous trigeminal thermorhizotomy in treatment of malignant facial pain. Acta Neurochir (Wien) 1983;69:283–9.
51. Mendelsohn D, Ranjan M, Hawley P, et al. Percutaneous trigeminal rhizotomy for facial pain secondary to head and neck malignancy. Clin J Pain 2013;29:e4–5.
52. Dar SA, Love Z, Prologo JD, et al. CT-guided cryoablation for palliation of secondary trigeminal neuralgia from head and neck malignancy. J Neurointerv Surg 2013;5:258–63.
53. Reddy GD, Viswanathan A. Trigeminal and glossopharyngeal neuralgia. Neurol Clin 2014;32:539–52.

Chronic/Persistent Idiopathic Facial Pain

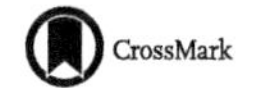

Joanna M. Zakrzewska, MD

KEYWORDS

• Facial pain • Persistent idiopathic facial pain • Cognitive behavior therapy • Antidepressants

KEY POINTS

- Persistent idiopathic facial pain is a poorly localized, often continuous nagging pain of the face for which no cause as yet has been identified.
- Patients are often overinvestigated in their quest to obtain a diagnosis and current conventional investigations are all normal.
- Systematic reviews highlight the paucity of randomized controlled trials of high quality with a combination of antidepressant and cognitive behavior therapy providing the best pain relief and decreased interference with life.
- A multidisciplinary biopsychosocial approach provides for the best outcomes, as these patients have significant comorbidities, including other chronic pain, personality disorders, and a history of significant life events.

INTRODUCTION

There has been considerable controversy about the condition currently called persistent idiopathic facial pain (PIFP) by the International Headache Society Classification (ICHD).[1] The term persistent as opposed to chronic is preferred, as it implies that relief may be a possible outcome. It is often called atypical facial pain (AFP).[2] In this text, both terminologies PIFP and AFP are used, but it is assumed that these are the same disorders. It may include more than one condition; for example, atypical odontalgia or persistent dentoalveolar pain. In the neurosurgical literature it has been termed AFP, and Burchiel[3] emphasized that it excludes disorders for which a cause has been identified and that this is a somatoform disorder diagnosed by psychological testing.

The ICHD description is "persistent facial and/or oral pain, with varying presentations but recurring daily for more than 2 hours per day over more than 3 months, in the absence of clinical neurologic deficit." See **Box 1** for criteria.

Box 1
International Headache Society Classification diagnostic criteria for persistent idiopathic facial pain

Diagnostic criteria

1. Facial and/or oral pain fulfilling criteria 2 and 3
2. Recurring daily for more than 2 hours per day for more than 3 months
3. Pain has both of the following characteristics:
   a. Poorly localized, and not following the distribution of a peripheral nerve
   b. Dull, aching or nagging quality
4. Clinical neurologic examination is normal
5. A dental cause has been excluded by appropriate investigations

Patients are diagnosed into this category frequently as an exclusion diagnosis; however, with improved appreciation of the need to take

Conflict of Interest: Known.
Division of Diagnostic, Surgical and Medical Sciences, Eastman Dental Hospital, UCLH NHS Foundation Trust, 256 Gray's Inn Road, London, WC1X 8LD, UK
E-mail address: j.zakrzewska@ucl.ac.uk

Neurosurg Clin N Am 27 (2016) 345–351
http://dx.doi.org/10.1016/j.nec.2016.02.012
1042-3680/16/$ – see front matter

careful history, patients who were previously put in this category may in fact have other identifiable causes of pain, such as neuropathic pain and myofascial pain, and so do not belong here.[4,5]

The cause remains unknown but it has been suggested that it could be a consequence of deafferentation and central sensitization but is still is not clear if peripheral or central mechanisms are involved.[4,6] Not surprisingly, psychological factors are identified but these also could be as a consequence of having chronic pain, lack of diagnosis, and attitude of health care professionals. Gustin and colleagues[7] have shown that psychological and psychosocial factors are universal to chronic pain and are no different between patients with orofacial pain relative to diagnosis.

EPIDEMIOLOGY

A study in primary care in the Netherlands found an incidence rate of 4.4 (95% confidence interval 3.2–5.9) for AFP with a predominance in women of 75% and mean age of 45.5 years (SD 19.6).[8] A review of 97 patients with facial pain attending a neurologic tertiary center in Austria classified 21% as having PIFP.[9] In a UK community-based study, chronic orofacial pain was identified in 7% of the population and these patients often have other unexplained symptoms, such as chronic widespread pain, irritable bowel syndrome, and chronic fatigue, and show high levels of health anxiety, reassurance-seeking behavior, and recent adverse events.[10]

Risk Factors

- Psychological distress
- Maladaptive response to illness
- Women
- Retrospective perception of unhappiness in childhood.[11,12]

On the other hand, in the large Finnish birth cohort study of 5696 individuals, a question on facial pain was added and a correlation was found with optimism, which was an important factor in reducing facial pain.[13]

Using the Chronic Graded Pain Scale, Chung and colleagues[14] showed, in a population study of elderly Koreans, that disability was high in nearly 50% of patients with chronic facial pain but lower than for other forms of facial pain, such as burning mouth and joint pain.

Major Predictors of Outcome

- Patients' illness beliefs such as serious consequences of continued pain
- Low personal control[15]
- Optimism[13]

CLINICAL FEATURES

If there is a history of trauma, extensive dental work before pain onset, for example, of 6 months, then the pain may be neuropathic and so should not be classified under this category. Trained staff may be able to establish a more accurate diagnosis that avoids the label of PIFP.[16] Taking a careful history, including family history, social history, and performing psychological testing, is imperative, as comorbidity is common.[17,18]

Table 1 lists the key features.

Pfaffenrath and colleagues[19] and Zebenholzer and colleagues[20] have both used the ICHD criteria to determine if the criteria are correct and both suggested alterations. Zebenholzer and colleagues[20] put forward very simple criteria for PIFP under which most chronic orofacial pain could be classified.

INVESTIGATIONS

Many of these patients will have had numerous investigations including MRIs and yet is it questionable whether they should have an MRI scan, as these are normal. Lang and colleagues[21] showed that patients with PIFP do not have neurovascular compression of their trigeminal nerve at the route entry zone. However, patients with PIFP have brain morphology changes consistent with those who have chronic pain,[22] but studies suggest that somatosensory processing is not used to maintain the pain.[23] Conditions such as temporal arteritis may need to be excluded in patients older than 50 years by appropriate investigations.

Table 1
Features of persistent idiopathic facial pain

Character	Dull, aching, nagging, sharp
Site and radiation	Deep, poorly localized, nonanatomic, intraoral, extraoral, change over time
Severity	Varying but can be intense
Duration and periodicity	Long, slow onset; continuous, intermittent
Provoking factors	Stress, fatigue
Relieving factors	Rest
Possible associated factors	Multiple other bodily pains Pruritus Dysmenorrhea Life events Personality disorders Anxiety, depression Sleep disturbance

Forssell and colleagues,[4] when comparing patients with trigeminal neuropathic pain with AFP, showed that up to 75% of patients with AFP demonstrated abnormalities on neurophysiological testing. If qualitative sensory testing and neurophysiological recordings are abnormal, this may result in changing the diagnosis to probable neuropathic pain.[5] It is important that these patients have some form of psychological testing, the easiest of which are psychometrically tested questionnaires such as the Brief Pain Inventory–Facial,[24] Hospital Anxiety and Depression Scale,[25] Pain Catastrophizing Scale,[26] and Chronic Graded Pain Scale.[27] These tests often show high levels of disability. A study of German University centers managing chronic facial pain showed that only 32% (6/19) did psychological testing.[9]

OVERALL MANAGEMENT

Often by the time these patients present in a specialist clinic they have been to numerous dentists and medical practitioners, attended at several secondary care centers, and had a significant number of investigations and some treatments that may have included irreversible dental treatments.[19] Studies in a German secondary care sector have shown inadequate management[9] and similar findings have been reported in the United Kingdom.[28] A qualitative study of doctors, dentists, and patients in the United Kingdom showed that current management of PIFP was ineffective and unsatisfactory from everyone's perspective.[29] The study identified especially relationships between clinician and patient and lack of psychological support.

Fig. 1 shows an algorithm used in a large UK facial pain clinic that is based on what evidence is currently available.

PHARMACOLOGIC TREATMENT OPTIONS

There are no high-quality evidence-based treatments. When List and colleagues[30] did a systematic review of pharmacologic treatments for facial pain they found very few studies and many of them were mixed, including both temporomandibular disorders and AFP. Probably the first trial was by Lascelles[31] in 1966, who used monoamine oxidase inhibitors in a crossover trial of 40 patients with PIFP and depression with some success.

Treatment is often specialty biased.[32] A survey among UK medical and dental practitioners

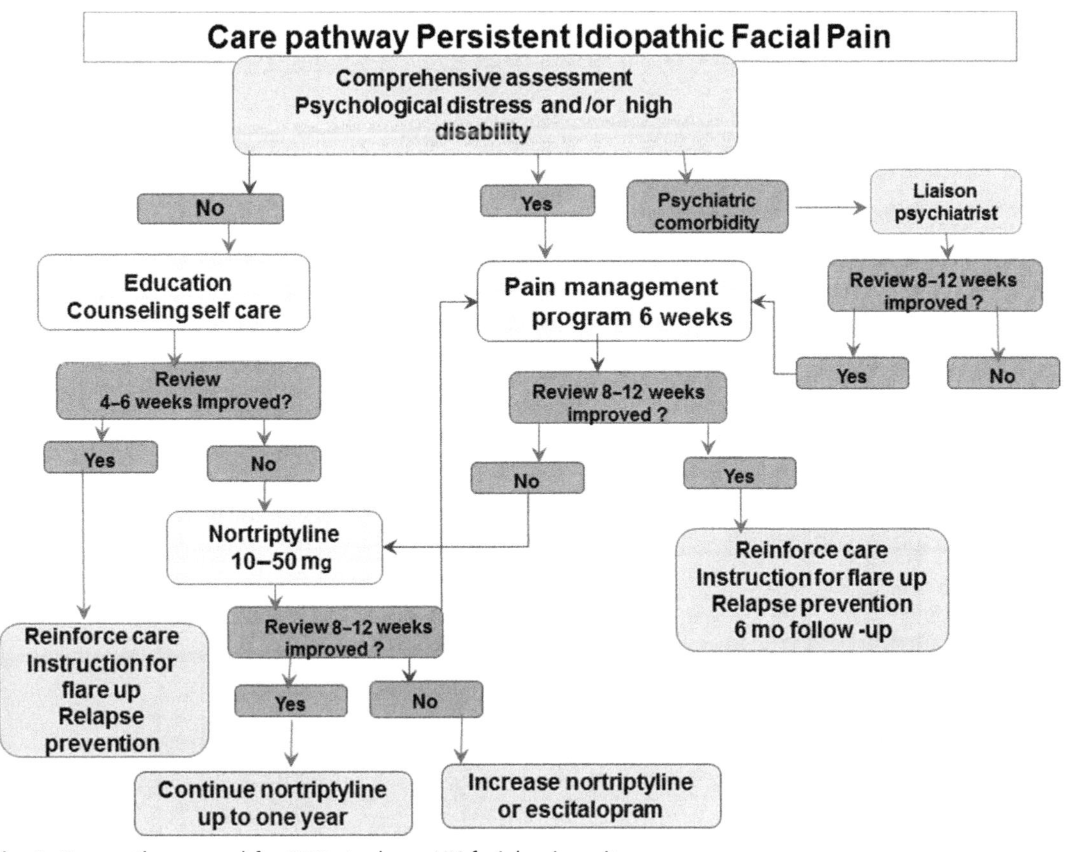

Fig. 1. Care pathway used for PIFP at a large UK facial pain unit.

Table 2
RCTs of drug treatments for persistent idiopathic facial pain

Drug	Trial Details	Efficacy	Side Effects	Comment	Reference
Venlafaxine 75 mg oral daily	RCT crossover, 2 wk each arm 30 patients	Modest on pain relief, 3 patients >30% pain reduction but not intensity, nil on anxiety depression	Little difference between placebo and active sweating and dryness	Underpowered and low dose of venlafaxine	Forssell et al,[44] 2004
Fluoxetine 20 mg Placebo CBT with or without fluoxetine	RCT 4 arms for 3 months 178 patients	Only fluoxetine on its own was effective in reducing pain intensity; addition of CBT reduced distress and level of interference; CBT on its own reduced interference only	None stated Largest dropout rate was in CBT	59 did not complete and some patients had TMD	Harrison et al,[40] 1997
Sumatriptan 6 mg Subcutaneous 1 dose	RCT crossover 1 d interval of 3–6 wk between crossover 19 patients	Temporary improvement, only 1 reported sustained relief	All reported side effects, headache, abnormal sensations	Assessed 60 and 120 min only	Harrison et al,[46] 1997 al Balawi et al,[45] 1996
Dothiepin 25–150 mg with biteguard, placebo and biteguard, dothiepin, placebo	RCT 4 parallel groups, 50 TMD, 43 AFP, 57 unclassified	Some pain relief with dothiepin but large dropout	Drowsiness, dry mouth, no details about withdrawals	Mixed cohort, inconclusive	Feinmann,[47] 1983

Abbreviations: AFP, atypical facial pain; CBT, cognitive behavior therapy; RCT, randomized controlled trial; TMD, temporomandibular disorder.
Data from Refs.[40,44–47]

showed that the most common drugs used were antidepressants.[2] Some selective serotonin reuptake inhibitors or selective noradrenalin and serotonin inhibitors are used.[33] Anticonvulsant drugs have not been shown to be effective.

Patients with significant psychiatric comorbidity will benefit from an assessment with a liaison psychiatrist before being referred to a cognitive behavior program.

Those studies that have been the subject of a randomized controlled trial (RCT) are shown in **Table 2**.

NONPHARMACOLOGIC TREATMENT OPTIONS

A systematic review of psychological therapies identified 17 trials in orofacial pain but there was a high risk of bias so only weak evidence was found to support their use.[34] A controlled patient-blinded study in 41 patients with PIFP compared active hypnosis for 5 1-hour individual sessions with relaxation and showed that significant pain relief was obtained in susceptible adults but there was a need for further psychological support to help with coping strategies and other psychological issues.[35]

It is crucial to stress that a cause cannot be found in all cases, and this does not mean that the pain is not real. Patients need to move away from looking for a cause and develop coping strategies, pacing, and targeting goals that would reduce interference with quality of life[36] and these sessions may be short.[37] Reassurance with an explanation is required rather than just a statement that "things will get better." Written patient information is helpful and these can be found on the European Federation Chapters http://efic.org/userfiles/Persistent_Idiopathic_Facial_Pain_EFIC.pdf, European Year against orofacial pain 2013/14. Techniques such as mindfulness, meditation, and yoga can be helpful. Sleep hygiene often needs to be improved, as poor sleep increases vulnerability to pain. These techniques are likely to have a positive outcome on other chronic pain, as cognitive behavior therapy has been shown to be effective in chronic pain.[38,39]

COMBINATION THERAPIES

Harrison and colleagues[40] showed that the best outcomes were obtained with a combination of an antidepressant with cognitive behavior therapy (see **Table 2**).

SURGICAL TREATMENT OPTIONS

In their series of 256 patients treated with Gamma Knife surgery, Balamucki and colleauges[41] included 20 patients with PIFP, and in this group, 60% had pain relief with 15% coming off all medication and up to 42% indicated that their quality of life had improved. However, there was a recurrence rate of 33%. Radiofrequency thermocoagulation or microvascular decompression gave satisfactory long-term pain relief in 16 patients.[42]

EVALUATION OF OUTCOME AND LONG-TERM RECOMMENDATIONS

There are few data on prognosis. Feinmann[43] followed patients who had undertaken a trial of dothiepin and at 4 years showed that improvement had been maintained, albeit with continuation of dothiepin, withdrawal at 6 months had resulted in return of pain. Long-term antidepressants may be needed as well as psychological support to reduce further health utilization.

SUMMARY/DISCUSSION

There remains little high-quality evidence on PIFP. Potentially this diagnosis is being used less often, as more detailed history and examinations are done that enable more accurate diagnosis; for example, neuropathic pain, burning mouth syndrome, and temporomandibular disorders. These patients have increased vulnerability to chronic pain and will present with many other medically unexplained symptoms and personality disorders. Their health utilization is high as they seek to obtain a diagnosis, exclude a serious cause for their disease, and then get treatment. They feel abandoned as once clinicians have excluded a serious or treatable cause they are reassured and discharged from clinics. Reassurance on its own is insufficient and it must be associated with written information and coping strategies. There is a paucity of high-quality trials confounded by the wide range of diagnostic criteria used. Some trials will include a variety of chronic orofacial pain conditions and do not report on them separately. A systematic review showed weak evidence for psychological therapy on its own but one RCT showed that when combined with antidepressants, improved outcomes are possible. PIFP is a long-term condition especially if not managed early, and patients need to be positively reassured that they are believed to have real pain but its cause currently remains unknown.

REFERENCES

1. Headache Classification Committee of the International Headache Society (IHS). The International Classification of Headache Disorders, 3rd edition (beta version). Cephalalgia 2013; 33(9):629–808.
2. Elrasheed AA, Worthington HV, Ariyaratnam S, et al. Opinions of UK specialists about terminology, diagnosis, and treatment of atypical facial pain: a survey. Br J Oral Maxillofac Surg 2004;42(6):566–71.
3. Burchiel KJ. A new classification for facial pain. Neurosurgery 2003;53(5):1164–6.
4. Forssell H, Tenovuo O, Silvoniemi P, et al. Differences and similarities between atypical facial pain and trigeminal neuropathic pain. Neurology 2007; 69(14):1451–9.
5. Forssell H, Jaaskelainen S, List T, et al. An update on pathophysiological mechanisms related to idiopathic oro-facial pain conditions with implications for management. J Oral Rehabil 2015;42(4):300–22.
6. Jaaskelainen SK, Forssell H, Tenovuo O. Electrophysiological testing of the trigeminofacial system: aid in the diagnosis of atypical facial pain. Pain 1999;80(1–2):191–200.
7. Gustin SM, Wilcox SL, Peck CC, et al. Similarity of suffering: equivalence of psychological and psychosocial factors in neuropathic and non-neuropathic orofacial pain patients. Pain 2011;152(4):825–32.
8. Koopman JS, Dieleman JP, Huygen FJ, et al. Incidence of facial pain in the general population. Pain 2009;147(1–3):122–7.
9. Wirz S, Ellerkmann RK, Buecheler M, et al. Management of chronic orofacial pain: a survey of general dentists in German university hospitals. Pain Med 2010;11(3):416–24.
10. Aggarwal VR, McBeth J, Zakrzewska JM, et al. The epidemiology of chronic syndromes that are frequently unexplained: do they have common associated factors? Int J Epidemiol 2006;35(2):468–76.
11. Macfarlane TV, Blinkhorn AS, Davies RM, et al. Oro-facial pain in the community: prevalence and associated impact. Community Dent Oral Epidemiol 2002;30(1):52–60.
12. Aggarwal VR, Macfarlane GJ, Farragher TM, et al. Risk factors for onset of chronic oro-facial pain–results of the North Cheshire oro-facial pain prospective population study. Pain 2010;149(2):354–9.
13. Sipila K, Ylostalo PV, Ek E, et al. Association between optimism and self-reported facial pain. Acta Odontol Scand 2006;64(3):177–82.
14. Chung JW, Kim JH, Kim HD, et al. Chronic orofacial pain among Korean elders: prevalence, and impact using the graded chronic pain scale. Pain 2004; 112(1–2):164–70.
15. Galli U, Ettlin DA, Palla S, et al. Do illness perceptions predict pain-related disability and mood in chronic orofacial pain patients? A 6-month follow-up study. Eur J Pain 2010;14(5):550–8.
16. Nobrega JC, Siqueira SR, Siqueira JT, et al. Differential diagnosis in atypical facial pain: a clinical study. Arq Neuropsiquiatr 2007;65(2A):256–61.
17. Sipila K, Ylostalo PV, Joukamaa M, et al. Comorbidity between facial pain, widespread pain, and depressive symptoms in young adults. J Orofac Pain 2006;20(1):24–30.
18. Feinmann C, Harris M, Cawley R. Psychogenic facial pain, presentation and treatment. Br Med J (Clin Res Ed) 1984;288:436–8.
19. Pfaffenrath V, Rath M, Pollmann W, et al. Atypical facial pain–application of the IHS criteria in a clinical sample. Cephalalgia 1993;13(Suppl 12):84–8.
20. Zebenholzer K, Wober C, Vigl M, et al. Facial pain and the second edition of the International Classification of Headache Disorders. Headache 2006; 46(2):259–63.
21. Lang E, Naraghi R, Tanrikulu L, et al. Neurovascular relationship at the trigeminal root entry zone in persistent idiopathic facial pain: findings from MRI 3D visualisation. J Neurol Neurosurg Psychiatry 2005;76(11):1506–9.
22. Schmidt-Wilcke T, Hierlmeier S, Leinisch E. Altered regional brain morphology in patients with chronic facial pain. Headache 2010;50(8):1278–85.
23. Lang E, Kaltenhauser M, Seidler S, et al. Persistent idiopathic facial pain exists independent of somatosensory input from the painful region: findings from quantitative sensory functions and somatotopy of the primary somatosensory cortex. Pain 2005; 118(1–2):80–91.
24. Lee JY, Chen HI, Urban C, et al. Development of and psychometric testing for the Brief Pain Inventory-Facial in patients with facial pain syndromes. J Neurosurg 2010;113(3):516–23.
25. Zigmond AS, Snaith RP. The hospital anxiety and depression scale. Acta Psychiatr Scand 1983;67: 361–437.
26. Sullivan MJ, Bishop SR, Pivik J. The pain catastrophizing scale: development and validation. Psychological Assessment 1995;7(4):524–32.
27. Von Korff M, Dworkin SF, Le Resche L. Graded chronic pain status: an epidemiologic evaluation. Pain 1990;40(3):279–91.
28. Beecroft EV, Durham J, Thomson P. Retrospective examination of the healthcare 'journey' of chronic orofacial pain patients referred to oral and maxillofacial surgery. Br Dent J 2013;214(5):E12.
29. Peters S, Goldthorpe J, McElroy C, et al. Managing chronic orofacial pain: a qualitative study of patients', doctors', and dentists' experiences. Br J Health Psychol 2015;20(4):777–91.
30. List T, Axelsson S, Leijon G. Pharmacologic interventions in the treatment of temporomandibular disorders, atypical facial pain, and burning mouth

syndrome. A qualitative systematic review. J Orofac Pain 2003;17(4):301–10.
31. Lascelles RG. Atypical facial pain and depression. Br J Psychiatry 1966;112(488):651–9.
32. Madland G, Feinmann C. Chronic facial pain: a multidisciplinary problem. J Neurol Neurosurg Psychiatry 2001;71(6):716–9.
33. Benoliel R, Eliav E. Neuropathic orofacial pain. Oral Maxillofac Surg Clin North Am 2008;20(2): 237–54, vii.
34. Aggarwal VR, Lovell K, Peters S, et al. Psychosocial interventions for the management of chronic orofacial pain. Cochrane Database Syst Rev 2011;(11):CD008456.
35. Abrahamsen R, Baad-Hansen L, Svensson P. Hypnosis in the management of persistent idiopathic orofacial pain–clinical and psychosocial findings. Pain 2008;136(1–2):44–52.
36. Madland G, Newton-John T, Feinmann C. Chronic idiopathic orofacial pain: I: what is the evidence base? Br Dent J 2001;191(1):22–4.
37. Harrison S, Watson M, Feinmann C. Does short-term group therapy affect unexplained medical symptoms? J Psychosom Res 1997;43(4):399–404.
38. Vlaeyen JW, Morley S. Cognitive-behavioral treatments for chronic pain: what works for whom? Clin J Pain 2005;21(1):1–8.
39. Morley S, Eccleston C, Williams A. Systematic review and meta-analysis of randomized controlled trials of cognitive behaviour therapy and behaviour therapy for chronic pain in adults, excluding headache. Pain 1999;80(1–2):1–13.
40. Harrison SD, Glover L, Feinmann C, et al. A comparison of antidepressant medication alone and in conjunction with cognitive behavioural therapy for chronic idiopathic facial pain. In: Jensen TS, Turner JA, Wiesenfeld Z, editors. Proceedings of the 8th World Congress on pain, progress in pain research and management. Seattle (WA): IASP Press; 1997. p. 663–72.
41. Balamucki CJ, Stieber VW, Ellis TL, et al. Does dose rate affect efficacy? The outcomes of 256 gamma knife surgery procedures for trigeminal neuralgia and other types of facial pain as they relate to the half-life of cobalt. J Neurosurg 2006;105(5):730–5.
42. Teixeira MJ, Siqueira SR, Almeida GM. Percutaneous radiofrequency rhizotomy and neurovascular decompression of the trigeminal nerve for the treatment of facial pain. Arq Neuropsiquiatr 2006;64(4): 983–9.
43. Feinmann C. The long-term outcome of facial pain treatment. J Psychosom Res 1993;37(4):381–7.
44. Forssell H, Tasmuth T, Tenovuo O, et al. Venlafaxine in the treatment of atypical facial pain: a randomized controlled trial. J Orofac Pain 2004; 18(2):131–7.
45. al Balawi S, Tariq M, Feinmann C. A double-blind, placebo-controlled, crossover, study to evaluate the efficacy of subcutaneous sumatriptan in the treatment of atypical facial pain. Int J Neurosci 1996;86(3–4):301–9.
46. Harrison SD, Balawi SA, Feinmann C, et al. Atypical facial pain: a double-blind placebo-controlled crossover pilot study of subcutaneous sumatriptan. Eur Neuropsychopharmacol 1997;7(2):83–8.
47. Feinmann C. Psychogenic facial pain: presentation and treatment. J Psychosom Res 1983; 27(5):403–10.

Future Directions for Surgical Trial Designs in Trigeminal Neuralgia

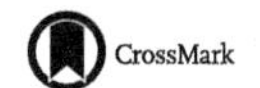

Joanna M. Zakrzewska, MD[a,*], Clare Relton, PhD[b]

KEYWORDS

• Research • Trial design • Randomized controlled trial • TN • Surgery • Cohort multiple RCT design

KEY POINTS

- There is no high-quality comparative effectiveness research for surgery versus pharmacologic management or for different surgical techniques.
- High-quality evidence (randomized controlled trials [RCTs]) is required to inform routine decision making for patients with trigeminal neuralgia (TN) and their consultants.
- The design and conduct of surgery trials using the standard design has numerous challenges (patient preferences, clinician preferences, clinically meaningful outcome measures, learning curves for surgical techniques, irreversibility of results).
- The "cohort multiple RCT" design is an innovative alternative design that provides both long-term observational data and a facility for quick and efficient conduct of multiple trials. Unlike standard trials, patient information and consent replicate that found in routine health care wherever possible.
- Embedding multiple trials within a cohort of patients with a diagnosis of TN would enable the quick and efficient identification and recruitment of patients to trials of a variety of interventions, and help provide the information that patients and clinicians require.

INTRODUCTION–WHICH TRIALS ARE NEEDED?

Unusually trigeminal neuralgia (TN), a rare disease, can be managed both medically (pharmacologically) and surgically, and there is some evidence of the importance of psychological therapies. So what trials are needed?

Comparison of Medical Versus Surgical Treatments

Surgical management can yield 100% pain relief for 70% of patients for 10 years.[1,2] Medical management provides 50% pain relief but becomes less effective over time, and as the dose is raised, results in poorer tolerability.[3] Many of these patients eventually opt for surgery, but the best timing for this is still unknown.[4] Although most patients remain on medical management until it fails,[5,6] there is evidence that *patients prefer surgical management*.[7] Zakrzewska and colleagues,[8] reviewing 220 patients who had posterior fossa, found 73% said they would have preferred earlier surgery.

There is also evidence that *clinicians/surgeons support early surgery* for classic cases of TN and those with positive imaging.[9] Others suggest that surgical treatments should be offered only after

Conflict of Interest: J.M. Zakrzewska has received consultancy fees from Convergence Pharmaceuticals Ltd. J.M. Zakrzewska undertook this work at UCL/UCLHT and received a proportion of funding from the Department of Health's NIHR Biomedical Research Center funding scheme.

[a] Division of Diagnostic, Surgical and Medical Sciences, Eastman Dental Hospital, UCLH NHS Foundation Trust, 256 Gray's Inn Road, London WC1X 8LD, UK; [b] School for Health and Related Research, University of Sheffield, Regent Court, 30 Regent Street, Sheffield S1 4DA, UK

* Corresponding author.

E-mail address: j.zakrzewska@ucl.ac.uk

Neurosurg Clin N Am 27 (2016) 353–363

http://dx.doi.org/10.1016/j.nec.2016.02.011

patients become refractory to medical management, which is defined by Obermann[10] as failure of 2 drugs. Di Stefano and colleagues[6] in their cohort of 200 patients on medical management suggest that medications remain highly effective and only 7% in their cohort needed surgery.

However, there is *no rigorous (ie, randomised controlled trial [RCT]) evidence to support either an early or delayed surgical management compared with pharmacologic management of TN*. The recent Cochrane systematic review on neurosurgical interventions in TN identified just 11 RCTs involving 496 patients[11]; however, most of these trials were biased. None of the high-quality trials compared different surgical techniques with each other or compared surgery with pharmacologic management. The 3 high-quality RCTs compared different surgical techniques with potentially more refined versions of the same technique.[11] There were no RCTs of microvascular decompression (MVD) (the most invasive procedure and only nondestructive procedure) but observational data suggests that it may have the best long-term outcomes for pain relief.[12]

Given patient and clinician preferences and the lack of evidence to support surgery or pharmacologic management, the most important research question for the TN profession is should patients undergo a surgical intervention as soon as the diagnosis has been made (ie, very early in the course of the condition), or should they wait until the conservative (pharmacologic) treatment has failed? In other words, should they receive surgical treatment that provides something very close to a cure (albeit not necessarily permanent) or remain on medication? If early surgery was comparable to (or better than) medical management, this information would affect how patients viewed their options at the time of diagnosis, and provide more flexibility in the decision-making process in the early stages.

Comparison of the Different Surgical Techniques

There are an emerging number of studies comparing different techniques; however, the interpretation of the results of these studies is hampered by differences in the outcomes used and the short duration of outcomes.[13] Future trials should use the same outcomes and also follow patients for a minimum of 5 years.[1]

New and Comparative Drug Trials

Drug trials in TN are few and far between and most drugs used to date have been established antiepileptics; however, there is now a potential for a new drug with good efficacy and better tolerability to be evaluated. Phase 2 studies have been completed using a novel design of enriched enrollment randomized withdrawal (EERW) design in which patients are initially screened, and then all are put on the active drug for a set period.[14] After this period, only those considered to have been responders are allocated to the randomized part of the trial in which the active drug is compared with a placebo. In this design, there is a set time for the trial but nonresponders are encouraged to drop out.

Moore and colleagues[15] have done a systematic review of all the pain trials using the EERW trial design and suggest that these can play an important role if correctly designed but may be difficult to compare outcomes with classic trials. Comparisons of different drugs are also required and whether single or multiple drugs should be used.[12]

Addition of Psychological Therapies

TN has considerable impact on quality of life and patients live in fear of a recurrence of their pain.[16] One small study (n = 15) has shown that spontaneous pain as opposed to pain evoked by a trigger could be driven by emotional factors.[17] There is anecdotal evidence from surgeons and patients that patients are reluctant to touch their faces after surgical treatments in case they trigger an attack. This behavior is also seen in continuation of medications after surgery, especially after stereotactic radiosurgery surgery (SRS).

In summary, there are a number of research questions in the field of TN that require evidence from well-designed RCTs. This article describes a number of challenges in the design and conduct of trials, with a particular emphasis on surgical trials for TN. It will provide some pointers for future trials.

PROBLEMS WITH RANDOMIZED CONTROLLED TRIALS

This section describes the problems with the design, implementation, and interpretation of RCTs of interventions to help patients with their health.

Recruitment

RCTs often have difficulty recruiting sufficient numbers of patients. MacDonald and colleagues[18] found that less than a third of 114 multicenter, publicly funded UK RCTs recruited their original target number of patients within the time originally specified. Failure to recruit to target may have implications for the power and generalizability of trial results. The sample populations often do not contain ethnic minorities or other hard-to-reach groups, for example, elderly individuals, making it difficult to apply to general practice. Trials of medical management in TN are all very small.[19]

Ethical issues

In a systematic review of the literature on barriers to participation in RCTs, Ross and colleagues[20] found that concerns with information and consent were some of the major reasons why both patients and clinicians were unwilling to participate in trials. In routine real-world health care, patients are rarely told of treatments that their clinicians cannot with certainty provide nor are patients told their treatment will be decided by chance.[21] On the other hand, in clinical trials providing this type of "full" information before randomization, is regarded as an ethical requirement. The consequence of this "full" information is that patients worry about the uncertainty of treatment outcome, especially if there is the possibility that they may be allocated to placebo. It is acknowledged that for clinicians there is a potential conflict of interest between what is good for the current patient and what is good for future patients.[22] These issues are nicely demonstrated in the anecdote in **Box 1**.

In a recent phase II trial, patients were reluctant to be recruited, as they had reasonable control and tolerability on their current drugs and were concerned that the new drug for TN would upset this balance (currently unpublished). Moreover, in general practice, patients are often given less information about their treatments than that currently required by some ethics committees who are asked to review intervention trials.

Box 1
Problems of informed consent

A Canadian surgeon participating in a workshop on designing clinical trials. The Canadian surgeon reported explaining a trial to a potential participant and the fact that there was uncertainty about the best treatment. At the end of the discussion the surgeon asked the patient if he had any questions. *"Yes"* said the patient, *"Can you refer me to a surgeon who does know what is the best treatment for me?"*

From Relton C. A new design for pragmatic randomised controlled trials: a 'Patient Cohort' RCT of treatment by a homeopath for menopausal hot flushes. [PhD thesis]. University of Sheffield; 2009.

Patient Preferences

Standard "open" (unblinded) pragmatic trials often compare an intervention with treatment as usual. Where the "usual care" on offer is available outside the trial, however, the only incentive for the patient to participate (apart from altruism) is to receive the new intervention. If a patient is allocated to treatment as usual, he or she may withdraw from the trial (attrition bias) or exhibit disappointment bias when reporting outcomes.[23] Patients with rare diseases are more reluctant to take part in trials for this reason.[24] There may therefore be a treatment effect, which results from patient preferences and not from therapeutic efficacy.[25] This is a major problem in TN, where destructive treatments give very different results from nondestructive methods or if compared with medical therapies. As surgery is irreversible, patients may prefer to delay this; yet, when asked specifically about timing of MVD most patients in retrospect said they would have wanted surgery earlier.[8]

Treatment Comparisons

For conditions with many potential treatment options, there are often multiple trials conducted, with each potential treatment being trialed, one at a time, in different populations by different research teams, often with heterogeneous outcomes and heterogeneous trial populations. Thus, when treatments need to be compared, they can only be done by indirect methods. The effectiveness of treatments A versus C can be difficult to evaluate if the only trials of treatments that exist are A versus B and B versus C. Indirect comparisons, in which 2 interventions are compared through their relative effect versus a common comparator, can succeed, but sometimes result in significant discrepancies compared with the results of head-to-head randomized trials.[26] Many competing interventions have thus not been compared or have been compared inaccurately, which is a waste of valuable information and money. This is a major problem in TN, where there are no RCTs of MVD and the RCTs that have been done compare surgical techniques and use varying outcome measures at varying time points. It has therefore been very difficult to compare not just surgical trials but medical trials for the same condition.

Diagnosis

An essential of all trials is an accurate description of the participants by using evidence-based diagnostic criteria, as this will enable clinicians to determine if the patients in the trial are representative of their patients. TN was considered to have very clear diagnostic criteria but it is now emerging that there are several variants and the nomenclature has become confusing with terms such as type 1 and 2 TN or TN with concomitant pain.[27,28] There has also been a group of conditions known as the trigeminal autonomic cephalalgias, which include 4 different conditions. Two of them, short unilateral neuralgiform headache with conjunctival redness tearing and short unilateral neuralgiform headache with any autonomic symptom, may in fact be yet other variants of TN.[29]

TN and its variants are unusual in that the pain is episodic and there are unpredictable remissions and relapses, which makes it even harder to be sure that the end result is due to the intervention rather than the natural history of the disorder.

Timing

New medications undergo a specific standardized pathway so as to become registered, but this is not the case for surgical interventions. A surgical intervention passes through many phases of innovation and refining and has a tipping point at which the intervention is no longer an innovation but a routine procedure. The tipping point (when equipoise is lost) is extremely variable and cannot be predicted, thus making the accurate timing of RCTs difficult.[30] This has generated what has become known as the Buxton law: "It is always too early [for rigorous evaluation] until suddenly it's too late."[21]

Thus, the newest intervention for TN, SRS, was first assessed in an exploratory trial to determine its efficacy and this was done in those patients who would benefit most and by surgeons who had the freedom to develop and refine the intervention. In 2001, an RCT by Flickinger and colleagues[31] of this procedure in a multicenter trial showed that 1 rather than 2 isocenters were sufficient to provide pain relief without sensory loss, one of the first refining studies. This could have been followed by a pragmatic trial that included a very broad population and surgeons with a range of expertise so it represented most closely what occurs in general practice. This approach would have provided information on both the short-term and long-term outcomes of SRS and could have addressed cost-effectiveness and quality-of-life questions if outcomes had been assessed independently.[23] This would have then enabled a standard to be set against which audits could be carried out. Schnurman and Kondziolka[32,33] have suggested an alternative approach to this problem (**Box 2**).

Box 2
The progressive scholarly acceptance (PSA) method

Aim:

- Use publications to chart progress from innovation to general acceptance.

Method:

- Assumes that once there is broad acceptance that an innovation is effective, the next series of papers focus on refining the technique.
- The point at which there are more papers on refinement than efficacy or effectiveness becomes the PSA point.
- Assess authoring group to see if the procedure was being disseminated and the quality of the publications.

Results:

- Refining studies increase efficiency, decrease costs, and may have a moderate effect on outcomes.
- Initial efficacy studies have a higher impact on patient care.

Schnurman and Kondziolka[33] then applied this to a series of surgical procedures, including SRS for TN. They found for this procedure 16 initial studies totally 1250 patients all of which were cohort ones and by 2002 there were 20 refining studies. The estimated year of progressive scholarly acceptance (PSA) was between 2002 and 2003 so objective efficacy i.e., time to acceptance by surgical community was 10 to 11 years. In comparison, endovascular coiling of aneurysms took only 5 years to objective efficacy. These results are also influenced by accessibility and approval of the equipment, the rarity of the disease, and the ease with which an RCT can be done. The investigators conclude that SRS for TN could be evaluated through an RCT.

Funding

Funding is often lacking, and estimates of costs of the studies can be difficult to predict due to the multiplicity of factors involved, and estimates become more complicated if the trials are multicentred.[34] Commercial influences often also come into play and may affect surgeons' involvement. The equipment for SRS is very expensive, and in cost evaluations, which also take into account quality-adjusted life years, SRS is the most expensive procedure of all surgical approaches.[35]

Choice of Comparators

There are many types of comparator available, but not all comparators are suitable for all types of surgery. Many trials compare surgical intervention with watchful waiting or medical treatment and this can be a satisfactory method for chronic conditions. When comparing surgical procedures, complications may be very different for the 2 interventions and this can affect both patient preference and blinding of outcomes; for example, ablative procedures are likely to result in sensory loss, whereas decompression of the trigeminal nerve is highly unlikely to lead to sensory loss but can result in hearing loss. When the comparator is a different surgical technique, then the same surgeon may be performing both interventions. He or she may be skilled in both but it is equally likely that there is a differential expertise between procedures. This then calls for a different approach that takes into account surgical expertise.[36] However, using expert surgeons may then result in an inability to generalize to all neurosurgeons.

Surgeons' Equipoise

Equipoise means that there is uncertainty regarding whether the trial treatment will be more beneficial to people than the comparator. Individual surgeons often have preferences for one intervention over another and thus may not be willing to take part in a clinical trial. Career surgeons are selected for traits that include comfort with making important clinical decisions quickly with incomplete information. This quality, required for decisive action during operations, may make it difficult for them to be consciously uncertain which of 2 treatments is better. Equipoise as to whether a treatment is effective or not is required in the scientific medical community but is not required from individual surgeons unless they have to perform 2 different types of surgical intervention in the trial. This can be a problem in neurosurgical interventions in TN, as some procedures are destructive, whereas others aim to preserve sensory function and so neurosurgeons may be reluctant to randomize patients to ablative procedures that they may consider using only in those patients who are not medically fit for major surgery.

Interventions

In pharmacologic trials, the main intervention in most cases is the drug alone; however, surgical interventions are highly complex and include the procedure itself, the surgeon, the surgical team, and preoperative and postoperative care.[9,15,23,37]

All surgical interventions have 2 learning curves, both of which are variable. The first is perfecting the surgical techniques and the second is the personal learning curve of the surgeon. This has been well illustrated when looking at the drop in mortality and complication rates of MVD for TN; over the years, mortality was more than 1% and now is approximately 0.2% to 0.4%.[38]

Blinding

Although it is considered important that both patients and health care professionals are blinded to ensure that exaggerated estimates of treatment are not reported, it can lead to patients being unsure of what is the required outcome and opting for an intermediate outcome.[39] However, this is much more difficult to do in nonpharmacologic trials than pharmacologic trials.[40] In a review of 110 RCTs evaluating treatment of pharmacologic and nonpharmacological interventions in patients with hip or knee osteoarthritis, it was shown that blinding was more difficult to achieve and unblinding occurred more frequently in nonpharmacologic intervention studies. Blinding of surgical procedures of patients/care providers is possible if the methods to blind are common. These include treatments that have the same physical characteristics and the same route of administration, surgical interventions that leave similar scars, and postoperative care; for example, number of isocenters for delivery of radiation to the trigeminal nerve but difficult to do when a using a frame or not for neuronavigation for delivery of radiofrequency thermocoagulation.[41] Blinding is improved if surgeons who performed the operation have no further contact with the patients. In studies in which treatments are radically different, for example, surgical versus drug therapy, or where control treatments are usual care or waiting list, then blinding of one group becomes impossible. In some trials, it may be easy to blind the patient to the procedure, but the subsequent clinical outcomes could result in unblinding; for example, different doses of radiation will lead to different complications. There is considerable evidence to show that unblinded outcomes assessment is associated with significantly larger treatment effects than blinded outcomes assessment.[42] When it is suspected that blinding may be problematic, it is useful to perform an assessment; for example, ask the patients which treatment they think they were given, as to whether the blinding was successful but current methods to do this assessment are far from standardized.[40]

Randomization

The strength of the RCT is that by randomization, assuming adequate concealment of group allocation, the distribution of any known or unknown prognostic factors at baseline arises purely by chance, thus randomization is the main method that ensures that allocation bias is eliminated at baseline.[30] It is often possible to randomize in the operating theater, as shown in the trial of Erdine and colleagues[43] of pulsed and continuous radiofrequency thermocoagulation for patients with TN. It is essential when analyzing the studies to ensure that the patients remain in the groups that they were randomized to at the beginning of the study; that is, use an intention-to-treat analysis.

Outcome Measures

Outcomes need to be varied and include clinical, patient-reported, and economic, both in the short-term and long-term. Developing valid reproducible generalizable outcome measures that are then suitable for meta-analysis is complex and requires considerable consensus. Boutron and colleagues[44] suggested a range of different types of outcome measures, which are listed in **Box 3**.

Different specialties have tried to develop some core outcome measures that will then lend themselves to meta-analysis and in determining the sample size of a study; for example, pain,[45] orthopedics.[46] Often some generic questionnaires are needed to compare to other data; the International Association for the Study of Pain has suggested a range of measures that should be used in clinical trials of pain patients (IMMPACT).[45] Measures using questionnaires need to undergo testing, which include its test-retest reliability (reproducibility), responsiveness (ability to detect clinically important change), and validity.[47] The major outcome measure of surgical treatments for TN has been pain relief, and there are very few reports of quality of life or other important patient outcomes.[48] The Barrow Neurologic Institute (BNI) scoring system[49] (which evaluates pain intensity and numbness) was first used in SRS and has been adopted by several centers. However, this has not undergone psychometric testing and it is not clear how it is administered; for example, from the medical notes or with the patient.[50] Reddy and colleagues[51,52] reported on the use of the BNI and a Visual Analog Scale to determine the minimum clinically important difference in pain improvement after an MVD[51] or SRS,[52] but the sample sizes were small. To overcome these shortcomings, Lee and colleagues[53] developed the Brief Pain Inventory Facial for which they also estimated the minimum clinically important differences[50] and have applied it before and after surgery to a group of patients undergoing SRS[54] and MVD.[55]

Box 3
Types of outcome measures

1. "Patient-reported outcomes" (eg, pain and disabilities), when the patient is the outcome assessor.
2. "Outcomes that do not suppose a contact between patients and outcome assessors" (eg, MRI).
3. "Outcomes that suppose a contact between patients and outcome assessors" (eg, sensory testing).
4. "Clinical events and therapeutic outcomes that will be determined by the interaction between patients and care providers" (eg, length of hospitalization, treatment failure, and repeat surgery), in which the care provider is the outcome assessor.
5. "Clinical events and therapeutic outcomes that will be assessed from data on the medical form" (eg, death, significant complication, short term, long terms). Boutron et al.

Poolman and colleagues[46] highlighted other difficulties in using outcome instruments; these include cultural and linguistic considerations, physical and mental capacity of patients, and the statistical methods used to evaluate them. Many outcome measures are in the form of questionnaires that then need to be administered in an independent way to prevent the assessor being blinded by the researcher; for example, patient completing questionnaire in the presence of or with help of the researchers.

Zarins[47] points out that in many trials the outcome measures are then applied in a modified form, which if they have not been tested invalidates them. Poolman and colleagues[46] showed in their review of outcome measures used in orthopedic RCTs that 10 trials (37%) used modified outcome measures and 9 did not describe how the modified instrument was validated and retested. Some questionnaires are generic and can be applied to a wide variety of conditions, for example, SF36, but can have little meaning for a specific entity. Thus, a questionnaire that has been validated for one clinical condition is not always valid when applied to a different clinical entity. Pan and colleagues[56] used the SF36 in their cohort of patients, but then did not find any other published study that used this tool and so went on to convert their data to the BNI, as they could then compare their data. The only validated questionnaires used in TN have been the verbal rating scale of pain, Hospital Anxiety and Depression Scale to measure mood, and the Brief Pain Inventory Facial for quality of life.

One of the major difficulties when comparing medical against surgical trials in TN is that for the latter, 100% pain relief is expected, whereas for drug management it is set at 50% in line with all other pain conditions. Patients' expectations of other outcomes may be different from medical versus surgical treatments.

FUTURE APPROACHES

Some important requirements of future trials are listed in **Box 4**.

There have been various attempts to address the difficulties in designing surgical trials. For example, the formation of the Balliol Colloquium, which reports its findings in a series of publications in the *Lancet*,[30,37,57] has put forward the IDEAL model of the stages in surgical practice, as shown in **Box 5**.

At all stages of the development of surgical practice, it is possible to use RCT designs. Although newer trial designs have been created to address some of the previously mentioned problems, none of these designs either increase the number of patients randomized and/or address the cost/funding problem with standard trials. More recently, a number of studies are embedding trials within cohorts as a way of overcoming these problems. These are described as follows.

TRIALS WITHIN COHORTS

Cohort Multiple Randomized Controlled Trial Design

In 2010, Relton and colleagues[58] published their theoretic article describing the "cohort multiple randomized controlled trial" design. This is an innovative approach to the design and conduct of pragmatic or comparative effectiveness trials, trials that aim to inform routine health care decision making.[58] The design aims to address many of the problems associated with standard RCT design that may reduce the generalizability of results, potentially introduce postrandomization selection bias, and create a suboptimal system for producing the information required for health care decision making. Since the publication of the theoretic article, a number of trialists have started using the design in the United Kingdom, Canada, and the Netherlands, including both trials with usual care as comparator; for example, trials within the PICNIC (prospective data collection initiative on colorectal cancer) cohort study of patients with rectal cancer (conference presentations). **Fig. 1** and **Box 6** illustrate how this may be used for TN.

Box 4
Requirements of future trials

- Use of multidisciplinary team and a range of different skills; for example, methodologists, statisticians, database designers, patients.
- Completion of a systematic review not only of clinical material but animal studies.
- Clinical trials protocol published before the trial start so they can be modified if necessary.
- All trials registered on trial sites, such as clinicaltrials.gov, before their completion so it is transparent that the protocol outcomes are used.
- The results published regardless of whether they are positive or negative. All randomized controlled trials (RCTs) should be reported using the CONSORT.

Box 5
Stages in IDEAL: innovation, development, exploration, assessment, and long-term study

- Stage 0: the initial pre-human work and development
- Stage 1 idea: first time it is used in human beings
- Stage 2a development: few patients recruited, few surgeons for the intervention
- Stage 2b exploration: early exploratory phase, reports appearing
- Stage 3 assessment: procedure is part of many surgeons' practices
- Stage 4 long-term study surveillance: databases set up, long-term outcomes, quality assurance

The rationale for this approach to informed consent is twofold. First, is that the primary motive for patients to enter clinical trials is not altruism, but their own direct benefit as patients. Clinical trial informed consent procedures should, therefore, put the needs of the patient at the center; that is, patients should not be told about treatments that they might not then receive, nor should they be told that their treatment will be allocated by chance. Second, the greater the similarity between patients' experiences in trials and their experiences in routine care, then the greater the generalizability of the trial results to patients in routine care.

The "cohort multiple RCT" design will not only yield much-needed data on long-term prognosis of this condition, but will allow both surgical and drug treatments and even adjunctive psychological treatments to all be evaluated alongside each other. It will also take into account patient and surgeon preferences, as it will be possible to evaluate the

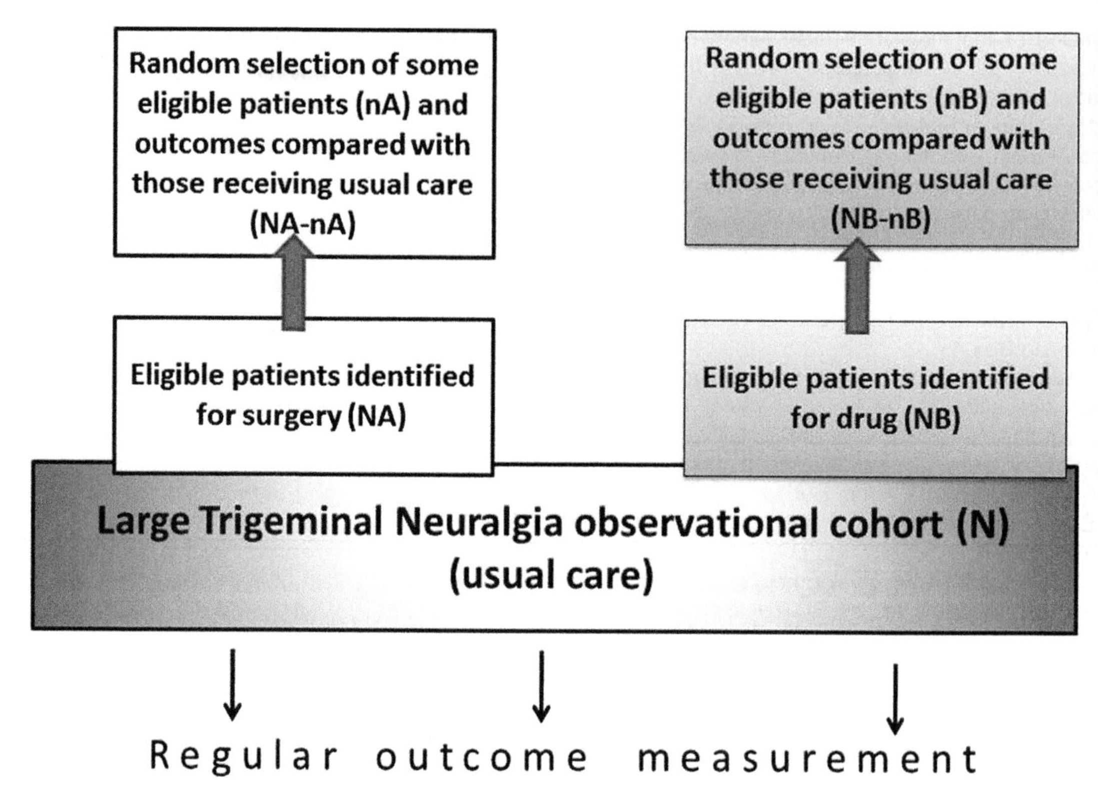

Fig. 1. A "cohort multiple RCT" approach to TN.

acceptability of different procedures by following those patients who refuse the offered RCT.

Research using standard RCT designs often struggles to recruit and consequently has to randomly allocate all patients to either group in equal proportions to maximize statistical power within their total sample. The large numbers of patients recruited to the cohort in the cmRCT approach increases the statistical power of any RCTs and enables unequal randomization. For example, a small number of patients could be randomly selected to be offered an expensive

Box 6
The key features of the "cohort multiple RCT" design

I. All patients with a diagnosis of trigeminal neuralgia (TN) are recruited into a large observational cohort study; all receive treatment as usual (which may include medical or surgical options).

II. Appropriate easily collected outcome measures are chosen and measured at regular intervals for the whole cohort, including description of treatment as usual.

For each RCT in the field of TN, for example, microvascular decompression, or a new drug.

III. All patients who are eligible for the trial are identified from the cohort "NA."

IV. Using randomization, a selection of patients "nA" are identified and then offered trial intervention "nA."

V. The outcomes of those randomly selected "nA" are then compared with the outcomes of those eligible patients not selected (but who were eligible to be selected) "NA-nA."

VI. The information given to patients and the consents sought from patients are as similar as possible to those found in routine care. All cohort patients consent to provide observational data at the outset; however, consent to "try" a particular intervention is sought only from those offered that intervention, thus replicating the patient-centered information and consent procedures that exist in routine health care, where clinicians provide patients with the information they need, at the time they need it.

treatment and compared with a larger number of unselected patients. Unequal randomization thus improves the efficiency of trials of high-cost interventions; for example, SRS, compared with equal allocation. These factors strengthen the inferences in the trial, lower treatment costs compared with standard designs (that is, once the cohort is established, it potentially allows for rapid and cheap recruitment of patients for any RCT), and allows significant cost savings for trials of expensive treatments. Furthermore, data on treatment refusers provides information on the acceptability of the treatment and thus the generalizability of the trial results.

Randomised Controlled Trial Within a Cohort Design

More recently, the cmRCT design has been adapted by the Finnish Degenerative Meniscal Lesion Study (FIDELITY)[59] to be able to incorporate one or more placebo trials of surgery within their cohort of patients with knee pain with meniscus injury. All patients recruited are informed that they may be offered a placebo intervention at some point. Sihvonen and colleagues[59] describe this as an "RCT within-a-cohort" design.

SUMMARY

This article has described some of the challenges encountered in trials and particularly surgical trials for TN, and provides some guidance for future trials. One future direction for TN research is to use designs that embed trials with cohorts, such as the innovative "cohort multiple RCT design." This approach enables multiple trials to be embedded within a single cohort of patients with TN, providing an efficient and effective approach to the testing of multiple interventions for TN with each other and with usual care.

REFERENCES

1. Tatli M, Satici O, Kanpolat Y, et al. Various surgical modalities for trigeminal neuralgia: literature study of respective long-term outcomes. Acta Neurochir (Wien) 2008;150(3):243–55.
2. Zakrzewska JM, Coakham HB. Microvascular decompression for trigeminal neuralgia: update. Curr Opin Neurol 2012;25(3):296–301.
3. Besi E, Boniface DR, Cregg R, et al. Comparison of tolerability and adverse symptoms in oxcarbazepine and carbamazepine in the treatment of trigeminal neuralgia and neuralgiform headaches using the Liverpool Adverse Events Profile (AEP). J Headache Pain 2015;16:563.
4. Zakrzewska JM, Linskey ME. Trigeminal neuralgia. BMJ 2014;348:g474.
5. Taylor JC, Brauer S, Espir MLE. Long-term treatment of trigeminal neuralgia. Postgrad Med J 1981;57:16–8.
6. Di Stefano G, La CS, Truini A, et al. Natural history and outcome of 200 outpatients with classical trigeminal neuralgia treated with carbamazepine or oxcarbazepine in a tertiary centre for neuropathic pain. J Headache Pain 2014;15:34.
7. Spatz AL, Zakrzewska JM, Kay EJ. Decision analysis of medical and surgical treatments for trigeminal neuralgia: how patient evaluations of benefits and risks affect the utility of treatment decisions. Pain 2007;131(3):302–10.
8. Zakrzewska JM, Lopez BC, Kim SE, et al. Patient reports of satisfaction after microvascular decompression and partial sensory rhizotomy for trigeminal neuralgia. Neurosurgery 2005;56(6):1304–11.
9. Nurmikko TJ, Eldridge PR. Trigeminal neuralgia–pathophysiology, diagnosis and current treatment. Br J Anaesth 2001;87(1):117–32.
10. Obermann M. Treatment options in trigeminal neuralgia. Ther Adv Neurol Disord 2010;3(2):107–15.
11. Zakrzewska JM, Akram H. Neurosurgical interventions for the treatment of classical trigeminal neuralgia. Cochrane Database Syst Rev 2011;(9):CD007312.
12. Cruccu G, Gronseth G, Alksne J, et al. AAN-EFNS guidelines on trigeminal neuralgia management. Eur J Neurol 2008;15(10):1013–28.
13. Zakrzewska JM, Linskey ME. Trigeminal neuralgia. BMJ 2015;350:h1238.
14. Zakrzewska JM, Palmer J, Ettlin DA, et al. Novel design for a phase IIa placebo-controlled, double-blind randomized withdrawal study to evaluate the safety and efficacy of CNV1014802 in patients with trigeminal neuralgia. Trials 2013;14:402.
15. Moore RA, Wiffen PJ, Eccleston C, et al. Systematic review of enriched enrolment, randomised withdrawal trial designs in chronic pain: a new framework for design and reporting. Pain 2015;156(8):1382–95.
16. Allsop MJ, Twiddy M, Grant H, et al. Diagnosis, medication, and surgical management for patients with trigeminal neuralgia: a qualitative study. Acta Neurochir (Wien) 2015;157(11):1925–33.
17. Moisset X, Villain N, Ducreux D, et al. Functional brain imaging of trigeminal neuralgia. Eur J Pain 2011;15(2):124–31.
18. MacDonald BK, Cockerell OC, Sander JW, et al. The incidence and lifetime prevalence of neurological disorders in a prospective community-based study in the UK. Brain 2000;123(Pt 4):665–76.
19. Zakrzewska JM, Linskey ME. Trigeminal neuralgia. BMJ Clin Evid 2014;2014.
20. Ross S, Grant A, Counsell C, et al. Barriers to participation in randomised controlled trials: a

systematic review. J Clin Epidemiol 1999;52(12): 1143–56.
21. Buxton MJ. Problems in the economic appraisal of new health technology: the evaluation of heart transplants in the UK. In: Drummond M, editor. Economic appraisal of health technology in the European Community. Oxford Medical Publications; 1987. p. 103–18.
22. Donnellan P, Smyth J. Informed consent and randomised controlled trials. J R Coll Surg Edinb 2001; 46(2):100–2.
23. Cook JA. The challenges faced in the design, conduct and analysis of surgical randomised controlled trials. Trials 2009;10:9.
24. Kesselheim AS, McGraw S, Thompson L, et al. Development and use of new therapeutics for rare diseases: views from patients, caregivers, and advocates. Patient 2015;8(1):75–84.
25. Torgerson DJ, Sibbald B. Understanding controlled trials. What is a patient preference trial? BMJ 1998; 316(7128):360.
26. Song F, Altman DG, Glenny AM, et al. Validity of indirect comparison for estimating efficacy of competing interventions: empirical evidence from published meta-analyses. BMJ 2003;326(7387):472.
27. Burchiel KJ. A new classification for facial pain. Neurosurgery 2003;53(5):1164–6.
28. Headache Classification Committee of the International Headache Society (IHS). The International Classification of Headache Disorders, 3rd edition (beta version). Cephalalgia 2013;33(9):629–808.
29. Lambru G, Matharu MS. SUNCT, SUNA and trigeminal neuralgia: different disorders or variants of the same disorder? Curr Opin Neurol 2014;27(3): 325–31.
30. Barkun JS, Aronson JK, Feldman LS, et al. Evaluation and stages of surgical innovations. Lancet 2009;374(9695):1089–96.
31. Flickinger JC, Pollock BE, Kondziolka D, et al. Does increased nerve length within the treatment volume improve trigeminal neuralgia radiosurgery? A prospective double-blind, randomized study. Int J Radiat Oncol Biol Phys 2001;51(2):449–54.
32. Schnurman Z, Kondziolka D. Evaluating innovation. Part 1: The concept of progressive scholarly acceptance. J Neurosurg 2016;124(1):207–11.
33. Schnurman Z, Kondziolka D. Evaluating innovation. Part 2: development in neurosurgery. J Neurosurg 2016;124(1):212–23.
34. Snowdon C, Elbourne DR, Garcia J, et al. Financial considerations in the conduct of multi-centre randomised controlled trials: evidence from a qualitative study. Trials 2006;7:34.
35. Sivakanthan S, Van Gompel JJ, Alikhani P, et al. Surgical management of trigeminal neuralgia: use and cost-effectiveness from an analysis of the Medicare Claims Database. Neurosurgery 2014;75(3): 220–6.
36. Devereaux PJ, Manns BJ, Ghali WA, et al. Physician interpretations and textbook definitions of blinding terminology in randomized controlled trials. JAMA 2001;285(15):2000–3.
37. Ergina PL, Cook JA, Blazeby JM, et al. Challenges in evaluating surgical innovation. Lancet 2009; 374(9695):1097–104.
38. Zakrzewska JM. Trigeminal neuralgia. In: Zakrzewska JM, Harrison SD, editors. Assessment and management of orofacial pain. 1st edition. Amsterdam: Elsevier Sciences; 2002. p. 267–370.
39. Day SJ, Altman DG. Statistics notes: blinding in clinical trials and other studies. BMJ 2000; 321(7259):504.
40. Boutron I, Estellat C, Ravaud P. A review of blinding in randomized controlled trials found results inconsistent and questionable. J Clin Epidemiol 2005; 58(12):1220–6.
41. Xu SJ, Zhang WH, Chen T, et al. Neuronavigator-guided percutaneous radiofrequency thermocoagulation in the treatment of intractable trigeminal neuralgia. Chin Med J (Engl) 2006;119(18):1528–35.
42. Poolman RW, Struijs PA, Krips R, et al. Reporting of outcomes in orthopaedic randomized trials: does blinding of outcome assessors matter? J Bone Joint Surg Am 2007;89(3):550–8.
43. Erdine S, Ozyalcin NS, Cimen A, et al. Comparison of pulsed radiofrequency with conventional radiofrequency in the treatment of idiopathic trigeminal neuralgia. Eur J Pain 2007;11(3):309–13.
44. Boutron I, Tubach F, Giraudeau B, et al. Blinding was judged more difficult to achieve and maintain in nonpharmacologic than pharmacologic trials. J Clin Epidemiol 2004;57(6):543–50.
45. Dworkin RH, Turk DC, Farrar JT, et al. Core outcome measures for chronic pain clinical trials: IMMPACT recommendations. Pain 2005;113(1–2):9–19.
46. Poolman RW, Swiontkowski MF, Fairbank JC, et al. Outcome instruments: rationale for their use. J Bone Joint Surg Am 2009;91(Suppl 3):41–9.
47. Zarins B. Are validated questionnaires valid? J Bone Joint Surg Am 2005;87(8):1671–2.
48. Akram H, Mirza B, Kitchen N, et al. Proposal for evaluating the quality of reports of surgical interventions in the treatment of trigeminal neuralgia: the Surgical Trigeminal Neuralgia Score. Neurosurg Focus 2013; 35(3):E3.
49. Rogers CL, Shetter AG, Fiedler JA, et al. Gamma knife radiosurgery for trigeminal neuralgia: the initial experience of The Barrow Neurological Institute. Int J Radiat Oncol Biol Phys 2000;47(4):1013–9.
50. Sandhu SK, Halpern CH, Vakhshori V, et al. Brief pain inventory–facial minimum clinically important difference. J Neurosurg 2015;122(1):180–90.
51. Reddy VK, Parker SL, Patrawala SA, et al. Microvascular decompression for classic trigeminal neuralgia: determination of minimum clinically

important difference in pain improvement for patient reported outcomes. Neurosurgery 2013; 72(5):749–54.
52. Reddy VK, Parker SL, Lockney DT, et al. Percutaneous stereotactic radiofrequency lesioning for trigeminal neuralgia: determination of minimum clinically important difference in pain improvement for patient-reported outcomes. Neurosurgery 2014; 74(3):262–6.
53. Lee JY, Chen HI, Urban C, et al. Development of and psychometric testing for the Brief Pain Inventory-Facial in patients with facial pain syndromes. J Neurosurg 2010;113(3):516–23.
54. Lee JY, Sandhu S, Miller D, et al. Higher dose rate Gamma Knife radiosurgery may provide earlier and longer-lasting pain relief for patients with trigeminal neuralgia. J Neurosurg 2015;123(4): 961–8.
55. Bohman LE, Pierce J, Stephen JH, et al. Fully endoscopic microvascular decompression for trigeminal neuralgia: technique review and early outcomes. Neurosurg Focus 2014;37(4):E18.
56. Pan HC, Sheehan J, Huang CF, et al. Quality-of-life outcomes after Gamma Knife surgery for trigeminal neuralgia. J Neurosurg 2010;113(Suppl): 191–8.
57. McCulloch P, Taylor I, Sasako M, et al. Randomised trials in surgery: problems and possible solutions. BMJ 2002;324(7351):1448–51.
58. Relton C, Torgerson D, O'Cathain A, et al. Rethinking pragmatic randomised controlled trials: introducing the "cohort multiple randomised controlled trial" design. BMJ 2010;340:c1066.
59. Sihvonen R, Paavola M, Malmivaara A, et al. Finnish Degenerative Meniscal Lesion Study (FIDELITY): a protocol for a randomised, placebo surgery controlled trial on the efficacy of arthroscopic partial meniscectomy for patients with degenerative meniscus injury with a novel 'RCT within-a-cohort' study design. BMJ Open 2013;3(3).

Surgical Options for Atypical Facial Pain Syndromes

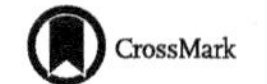

Shervin Rahimpour, MD, Shivanand P. Lad, MD, PhD*

KEYWORDS

- Atypical facial pain • Nucleus caudalis • DREZ • Motor cortex stimulation

KEY POINTS

- Atypical facial pain is often recalcitrant to pharmacotherapy; appropriate patient selection can make surgery a viable and appropriate option for treatment.
- Nucleus caudalis dorsal root entry zone lesioning is an effective and safe means of treating atypical facial pain.
- Motor cortex stimulation is an alternative intervention to consider for patients who do not respond to nucleus caudalis dorsal root entry zone lesioning.

INTRODUCTION

Facial pain syndromes encompass a body of diagnoses that can fit a very defined and classic presentation to one that is murkier and not localizable by physical examination or radiographic imaging. Beyond typical trigeminal neuralgia, atypical subtypes are often difficult to treat and refractory to common interventions. Herein, the *atypical subtype* is used as a catchall phrase to define trigeminal pain, not defined by trigeminal neuralgia type I or II by the Burchiel classification (**Table 1**).[1] The current spectrum of treatment of these syndromes includes pharmaceutical therapy, percutaneous procedures (chemical, thermal, irradiative, mechanical destruction), as well as open surgery, which includes microvascular decompression (MVD) and less often peripheral nerve stimulation, motor cortex stimulation, neurectomy, tractotomy, and nucleus caudalis dorsal root entry zone (NC DREZ) lesioning, though there is currently no mutual understanding of terminology, diagnosis, or treatment of facial pain[2] (**Table 2**). Several treatment algorithms have been developed for the treatment of facial pain with these various modalities.[3–6] Alksne and colleagues[6] used preoperative risk assessment and the presence of a vascular loop on MRI imaging for the treatment of trigeminal neuralgia with MVD versus Gamma Knife radiosurgery. In the single-institution experience by Munawar and colleagues[3] atypical subtypes as well as less-often-used treatment modalities are incorporated in a more comprehensive treatment algorithm. Specifically, treatment with tractotomy is considered only in cases of cancer facial pain. Neurectomy and motor cortex stimulation are used in cases of trigeminal neuropathic pain and deafferentation-type injuries. Of note, NC DREZ lesioning is considered less often and thought to be a more morbid and invasive procedure. Since

Disclosure Statement: S.P. Lad has consulted for and received grant support from Medtronic, Boston Scientific, and St. Jude Medical. None of the above contributed to the writing of the article, payment, or decision to submit for publication. He serves as Director of the Duke Neuro-Outcomes Center, which has received research funding from NIH KM1 CA 156687, Medtronic Inc, and St. Jude Medical. The remaining author reports no conflicts of interest.
Department of Neurosurgery, Duke University Medical Center, DUMC 3807, Durham, NC 27710, USA
* Corresponding author.
E-mail address: nandan.lad@dm.duke.edu

Neurosurg Clin N Am 27 (2016) 365–370
http://dx.doi.org/10.1016/j.nec.2016.02.010
1042-3680/16/$ – see front matter

Table 1
Burchiel classification scheme for facial pain

	Pain Category	History
Typical	Trigeminal neuralgia (type 1)	<50% episodic, typical trigeminal pain
	Trigeminal neuralgia (type 2)	>50% constant, typical trigeminal pain
Atypical	Trigeminal neuropathic pain	Unintentional injury secondary to dental/sinus injury, craniofacial trauma
	Trigeminal deafferentation pain (anesthesia dolorosa)	Intentional deafferentation secondary to destructive procedure
	Symptomatic trigeminal neuralgia	Multiple sclerosis, mass lesion (posterior fossa lesion)
	Postherpetic neuralgia	Herpes zoster (trigeminal distribution)
	Atypical facial pain	Somatoform pain disorder

Adapted from Burchiel KJ. A new classification for facial pain. Neurosurgery 2003;53(5):1166; with permission.

1982, NC DREZ lesioning at Duke has been refined to become safer and less invasive.[7–9] Furthermore, patient outcomes in the Nashold experience were reassuring with 96% pain relief postoperatively and 67% even still at 1 year. Patients were treated for postherpetic neuralgia, deafferentation pain (anesthesia dolorosa, post-tic dysesthesia, stroke, multiple sclerosis, gasserian tumor, Gamma Knife radiation injury), facial trauma/surgery, atypical facial pain, and migraine/cluster headache with success. More recently, Chivukula and colleagues[10] reported 75% improvement in quality of life and greater than 50% pain reduction at the 8-year follow-up (16 patients). Therefore, the authors emphasize NC DREZ for the treatment of these atypical subtypes, a procedure the authors think is underused and, in their cohort, proven to be very effective.

Table 2
Summary of current procedures for treatment of facial pain

	Procedure	Details	Notes
First order neurons	Microvascular decompression	Retrosigmoid craniectomy and vascular decompression of offending vessel from trigeminal nerve root	Nondestructive, complications include cerebrospinal fluid leak and vascular injury though routine procedure, widely accepted
	Destructive lesioning	Percutaneous needle insertion; chemical (glycerol), thermal (radiofrequency), or mechanical (balloon) destruction of trigeminal nerve	Destructive, does not require general anesthesia, can be selective for pain distribution, may result in numbness or dysesthesia, immediate pain relief
	Stereotactic radiosurgery	Stereotactic radiation of trigeminal nerve root	Destructive, noninvasive, may take several months for symptom relief
	Peripheral nerve stimulation	Peripheral trigeminal nerve electric stimulation	Nondestructive, trial period before permanent placement, adjustable settings for optimization
Second order neurons	NC DREZ lesioning	Radiofrequency ablation of nucleus caudalis from a posterior midline approach	Destructive, invasive, risk of transient ipsilateral limb ataxia
Third order neurons	Motor cortex stimulation	Epidural stimulation of motor cortex through burr hole	Nondestructive, invasive requiring craniotomy, adjustable settings for optimization

Adapted from Slavin KV, Nersesyan H, Colpan ME, et al. Current algorithm for the surgical treatment of facial pain. Head Face Med 2007;3:30.

With this experience in mind, the authors consider a new treatment algorithm for the treatment of atypical facial pain.

Diagnosis and Anatomy

Standard inclusion and exclusion criteria do not exist for either NC DREZ or motor cortex stimulation. A comprehensive physical examination, history, and evaluation both by a pain neurologist and psychologist (to exclude somatoform disorder) are necessary for the workup of chronic recalcitrant facial pain.[11] Typical trigeminal neuralgia is often described as episodic, sharp, and shocklike in the trigeminal distribution occurring in bursts either less than 50% (type 1) or greater than 50% (type 2) of the time, triggered by non-noxious stimuli, such as speaking, eating, or brushing teeth.[12] Atypical facial pain, on the other hand, is different in quality, more often described as constant, burning, throbbing, and aching facial pain. Furthermore, this type of pain is characteristically unresponsive to anticonvulsant drugs. At the time of surgical consideration, other causes, such as typical trigeminal neuralgia and headache, must be ruled out. Finally, psychological evaluation and testing is imperative.

Anatomically, trigeminal afferents (*primary neurons*) carrying pain and temperature fibers enter the pons and bifurcate, sending a caudal branch into the medulla, known as the descending trigeminal tract. At the level of the cervicomedullary junction, the spinal trigeminal nucleus overlies the descending tract. This tract also carries with it sensory fibers from the 7th, 9th, and 10th cranial nerves. The trigeminal afferents are topographically separated into 3 subdivisions (rostral to caudal): nucleus oralis, nucleus interpolaris, and nucleus caudalis located at the cervical medullary junction extending down to the level of C2. *Secondary neurons* then go on to synapse in the ventroposteromedial nucleus before *tertiary neurons* terminate at the level of the somatosensory cortex. Deafferentation injury is thought to lead to spontaneous signaling of secondary neurons leading to central facial pain. In this article, the authors consider therapies that target nociceptive signaling at the level of the trigeminal nucleus caudalis (NC DREZ), extending to the somatosensory cortex (motor cortex stimulation). Furthermore, the authors differentiate therapies as those targeting primary neurons (MVD, destructive lesioning, stereotactic radiosurgery), secondary neurons (NC DREZ), and tertiary neurons (motor cortex stimulation) of the trigeminal pain pathway.

Surgical Options

Nucleus caudalis dorsal root entry zone lesioning

Ablation of the trigeminal pain pathway by way of tractotomy-nucleotomy or by open surgical NC DREZ lesioning has been shown to be an effective means of treating atypical facial pain. First operated on by Sjöquist, several modifications have been made since to trigeminal tract surgery.[13,14] Typically, tractotomy and nucleotomy are considered before NC DREZ. Although the data comparing these procedures are limited, reported benefits for NC DREZ seem to be superior to tractotomy and nucleotomy for facial pain. Specifically, NC DREZ is effective for postherpetic neuralgia and craniofacial pain conditions and has also been used for chronic cluster headache, vagal or glossopharyngeal neuralgias, and intractable pain syndromes secondary to cancer/craniofacial surgery/trauma. This is because pain fibers from not only the area of the trigeminal nerve but also the facial, glossopharyngeal, and vagus cranial nerves synapse in second order neurons in the nucleus caudalis. The procedure uses the fact that pain- and temperature-carrying fibers separate from motor and touch sensation at the pons, therefore, allowing selective ablation. These first order neurons descend as part of the descending trigeminal tract and synapse to secondary neurons of the nucleus caudalis where it is thought spontaneous pain generation occurs in the case of deafferentation injury.

NC DREZ can use computed tomography (CT)–guided stereotactic navigation as first described by Kanpolat and colleagues[13] for tractotomy. A mini vertical midline incision is centered over the foramen magnum and dissected down to the C1 arch to ultimately expose dura. With the cord exposed (**Fig. 1**), relevant anatomy can be visualized, including the

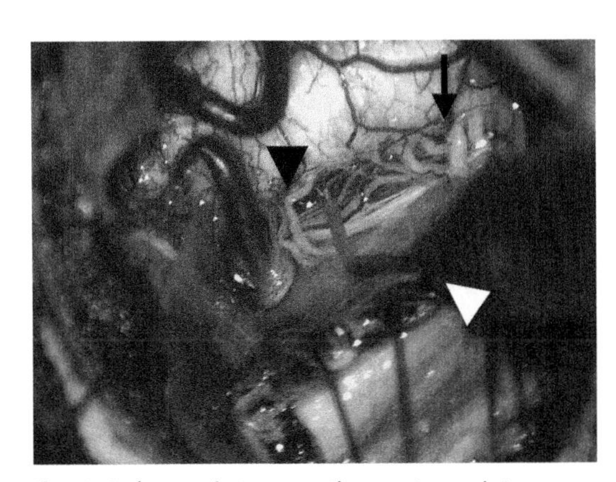

Fig. 1. Relevant intraoperative anatomy. Intraoperative imaging demonstrating relevant anatomy. Electrode (*white arrowhead*), accessory nerve rootlets (*black arrow*), and C2 nerve roots (*black arrowhead*).

vertebral artery, posterior inferior cerebellar artery, as well as the accessory nerve rootlets, C1/C2 roots, and pial vessels. Endoscopic assistance is also used for further visualization of anatomy beyond the extent of our exposure. Somatosensory-evoked potentials are then used to ensure trigeminal afferents are targeted as well as motor evoked potentials to ensure absence of the corticospinal tract. Given the proximity of the accessory nerve rootlets, trapezius stimulation can be seen. Once anatomic and electrographic anatomy is ensured, lesions are made to the nucleus caudalis extending from the obex to the level of the C2 nerve root. Between 1982 and 1988, in its first iteration, NC DREZ lesioning resulted in transient ipsilateral limb ataxia as a result of damage to the neighboring spinocerebellar tract. These side effects of the procedure eventually resolved but led to the second phase of the procedure with new electrode design incorporating insulation near the tip, which spared the spinocerebellar tract. Finally third-generation electrodes were developed to account for nucleus caudalis anatomy. Specifically, the cephalad nucleus caudalis is larger (~2 mm) and, below the level of C1, diminishes in size and becomes elongated and elliptical. As a result, 2 electrode tips were developed to lesion a deeper/wider nucleus caudalis at the level of the obex and a shallower/narrower nucleus caudalis between C1 and C2.[15] Finally, in its current form, the authors have used CT/MRI guidance, trigeminal neuromonitoring, and a minimally invasive endoscopic-assisted lesioning. A post-operative MRI is shown in **Fig. 2**, demonstrating the area of lesioning.

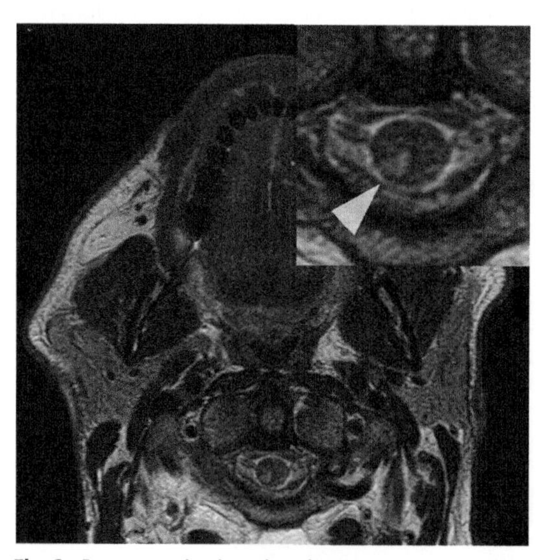

Fig. 2. Postoperative imaging demonstrating NC DREZ lesioning at one level. Postoperative axial T2-weighted imaging following NC DREZ lesioning. *Arrowhead* indicates the site of lesioning.

The authors' experience at Duke over the last 3 decades with NC DREZ has been positive. With greater than 70% pain relief, transient complications, and very high patient satisfaction, the authors treat atypical facial pain syndromes with DREZ lesioning as opposed to peripheral nerve stimulation, neurectomy, and motor cortex stimulation. Given its minimal invasiveness, safety, and reproducibility, the authors also advocate for its consideration as a therapeutic option for these challenging conditions refractory to other medical and interventional therapies.

Motor cortex stimulation

Penfield first demonstrated the idea that cortical stimulation can produce analgesia in the 1930s.[16] Not until 1991 did Tsubokawa and colleagues[17] formally describe motor cortex stimulation as a treatment of facial pain. Mechanistically, it is thought that motor cortex stimulation restores highly organized reciprocal pathways between primary motor and somatosensory cortex (layer I), and it is known that the somatosensory cortex can attenuate nociceptive signals.[18,19] Deafferentation injuries can disrupt this attenuation leading to aberrant connections; therefore, nonpainful stimuli elicit severe pain.[20] Other mechanisms suggest activation of functional networks involving the anterior cingulate cortex, orbitofrontal cortex, medial thalamus, and periaqueductal gray (PAG).[19,21] Finally, some evidence suggests that motor cortex stimulation increases secretion of endogenous opioids particularly in the anterior middle cingulate cortex as well as PAG.[22] Although motor cortex stimulation seems to alleviate deafferentation injury–related pain, no standard inclusion or exclusion criteria exist for treatment.

The procedure entails introduction of an electrode following burr hole placement. This procedure is done epidurally, though subdural lead placement has also been described. Image-guided neuronavigation is also used to ensure that the lead is placed over the premotor and precentral gyrus. Since its initial inception, a limited number of studies have described the efficacy of this procedure in a variety of pain syndromes, including poststroke pain, phantom-limb pain, postherpetic neuralgia, and other neuropathic facial pain syndromes. In fact, of these studies, 75% to 100% of patients reported good or excellent pain relief.[23–25] Specifically, in a study by Ebel and colleagues,[24] 7 patients with trigeminal neuropathic pain (dysesthesia, anesthesia dolorosa, and postherpetic neuralgia) underwent motor cortex stimulation. In all but one patient, a successful test stimulation period led to permanent lead placement. Of those patients, 50% maintained excellent pain control at the 5-month to 2-year follow-ups. A subsequent and more comprehensive

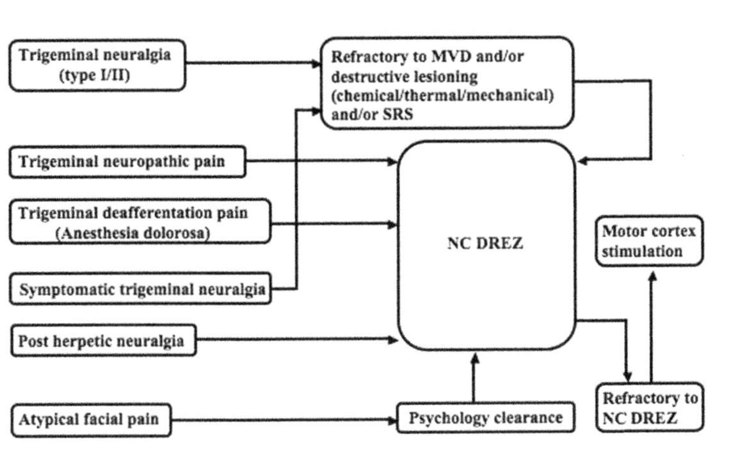

Fig. 3. Proposed atypical facial pain treatment algorithm.

report of 10 patients by Brown and Pilitsis[26] again showed that 7 of 8 patients who underwent permanent lead placement had immediate pain relief postoperatively of 50% or greater. Seventy-five percent of these patients continued to have sustained pain relief at the 3- to 24-month follow-up. A more recent review of the literature identified 118 patients with chronic neuropathic facial pain treated with motor cortex stimulation.[27] Of these cases, 84% continued to have good pain relief by the end of their study period. Of the whole reviewed group, the most common complication was seizure followed by wound infection. Of note, 2 patients treated by Henderson and colleagues[28] were able to recapture the benefit of motor cortex stimulation with reprogramming of the stimulator parameters. In fact, a review of these stimulation parameters showed a wide variety of rate (hertz), pulse width (microseconds), and amplitude (milliampere), without a clear consensus.[29] Therefore, although motor cortex stimulation has been shown to be effective in managing patients with common treatment-refractory neuropathic facial pain, there may be room for even further improvement by optimizing stimulation parameters.

Other surgical interventions

Tractotomy and nucleotomy, first described in 1938, targets facial pain at the tractus at the cervicomedullary junction.[14] In a series of 17 patients, Kanpolat and colleagues[30] performed this procedure with excellent pain relief in 44% and moderate pain relief in 56% of patients. One patient remained with pain and underwent NC DREZ, with subsequent resolution of pain relief up to the 2-year follow-up. Given the minimally invasive nature of the procedure, it was, therefore, advocated that patients undergo tractotomy-nucleotomy before NC DREZ is considered.

Since its inception in the middle of the twentieth century, deep brain stimulation of the thalamus and caudate has also been used in the treatment of chronic pain.[31] However, results of 2 multicenter trails were unfortunately inconclusive.[32] Several stimulation targets have been used, including PAG, zona incerta, and the ventral posterolateral nucleus of the thalamus. In a recent double-blinded study by Rasche and colleagues[33] of 56 patients with neuropathic pain, 6 patients had trigeminal neuropathic pain. Of these patients, half, at 30 months of mean follow-up, had an unsatisfactory response to the treatment. Deep brain stimulation, however, remains a poorly understood intervention for neuropathic pain; much remains to be learned about its role in the facial pain treatment algorithm.

SUMMARY

Currently there is no consensus on the treatment of atypical facial pain. In the authors' experience and a cohort of patients with difficult-to-treat facial pain, they have found NC DREZ to be an effective and safe procedure that is underused in this patient population. Therefore, the authors advocate for a treatment algorithm as outlined in **Fig. 3**. This procedure has been refined at Duke to be less invasive, safer, and as a result used more routinely. Lastly, the authors also use motor cortex stimulation as an option for patients refractory to other interventions. These two surgical interventions have been effective and safe in the treatment of facial pain syndromes refractory to conventional interventions, including MVD and percutaneous procedures, though certainly subsequent validation studies will be needed.

REFERENCES

1. Burchiel KJ. A new classification for facial pain. Neurosurgery 2003;53(5):1164–6 [discussion: 1166–7].
2. Elrasheed AA, Worthington HV, Ariyaratnam S, et al. Opinions of UK specialists about terminology,

diagnosis, and treatment of atypical facial pain: a survey. Br J Oral Maxillofac Surg 2004;42(6):566–71.
3. Munawar KV, Nersesyan H, Colpan ME, et al. Current algorithm for the surgical treatment of facial pain. Head Face Med 2007;3:30.
4. Amirnovin R, Neimat JS, Roberts JA, et al. Multimodality treatment of trigeminal neuralgia. Stereotact Funct Neurosurg 2005;83(5–6):197–201.
5. Stidd DA, Wuollet AL, Bowden K, et al. Peripheral nerve stimulation for trigeminal neuropathic pain. Pain Physician 2012;15(1):27–33.
6. Alksne HE, Nakaji P, Lu DC, et al. Multimodality treatment of trigeminal neuralgia: impact of radiosurgery and high resolution magnetic resonance imaging. J Clin Neurosci 2006;13(2):239–44.
7. Bullard DE, Nashold BS. The caudalis DREZ for facial pain. Stereotact Funct Neurosurg 1997; 68(1–4 Pt 1):168–74.
8. Gorecki JP, Nashold BS. The Duke experience with the nucleus caudalis DREZ operation. Acta Neurochir Suppl 1995;64:128–31.
9. Bernard EJ, Nashold BS, Caputi F, et al. Nucleus caudalis DREZ lesions for facial pain. Br J Neurosurg 1987;1(1):81–91.
10. Chivukula S, Tempel ZJ, Chen C-J, et al. Spinal and nucleus caudalis dorsal root entry zone lesioning for chronic pain: efficacy and outcomes. World Neurosurg 2015;84(2):494–504.
11. Zakrzewska JM. Differential diagnosis of facial pain and guidelines for management. Br J Anaesth 2013;111(1):95–104.
12. Haviv Y, Khan J, Zini A, et al. Trigeminal neuralgia (part I): revisiting the clinical phenotype. Cephalalgia 2015. http://dx.doi.org/10.1177/0333102415611405.
13. Kanpolat Y, Savas A, Batay F, et al. Computed tomography-guided trigeminal tractotomy-nucleotomy in the management of vagoglossopharyngeal and geniculate neuralgias. Neurosurgery 1998;43(3):484.
14. Sjöqvist O. Studies on pain conduction in trigeminal nerve: a contribution to the treatment of facial pain. Acta Psychiatr Neurol 1938;17(suppl):1–139.
15. Nashold BS, el-Naggar AO, Ovelmen-Levitt J, et al. A new design of radiofrequency lesion electrodes for use in the caudalis nucleus DREZ operation. Technical note. J Neurosurg 1994;80(6):1116–20.
16. Lende RA, Kirsch WM, Druckman R. Relief of facial pain after combined removal of precentral and postcentral cortex. J Neurosurg 1971;34(4):537–43.
17. Tsubokawa T, Katayama Y, Yamamoto T, et al. Chronic motor cortex stimulation for the treatment of central pain. Acta Neurochir Suppl (Wien) 1991;52:137–9.
18. Canavero S, Bonicalzi V. Therapeutic extradural cortical stimulation for central and neuropathic pain: a review. Clin J Pain 2002;18(1):48–55.
19. Brown JA, Barbaro NM. Motor cortex stimulation for central and neuropathic pain: current status. Pain 2003;104(3):431–5.
20. Loeser JD, Ward AA, White LE. Chronic deafferentation of human spinal cord neurons. J Neurosurg 1968;29(1):48–50.
21. Peyron R, Garcia-Larrea L, Deiber MP, et al. Electrical stimulation of precentral cortical area in the treatment of central pain: electrophysiological and PET study. Pain 1995;62(3):275–86.
22. Maarrawi J, Peyron R, Mertens P, et al. Motor cortex stimulation for pain control induces changes in the endogenous opioid system. Neurology 2007;69(9):827–34.
23. Nguyen JP, Keravel Y, Feve A, et al. Treatment of deafferentation pain by chronic stimulation of the motor cortex: report of a series of 20 cases. Acta Neurochir Suppl 1997;68:54–60.
24. Ebel H, Rust D, Tronnier V, et al. Chronic precentral stimulation in trigeminal neuropathic pain. Acta Neurochir (Wien) 1996;138(11):1300–6.
25. Meyerson BA, Lindblom U, Linderoth B, et al. Motor cortex stimulation as treatment of trigeminal neuropathic pain. Acta Neurochir Suppl (Wien) 1993;58: 150–3.
26. Brown JA, Pilitsis JG. Motor cortex stimulation for central and neuropathic facial pain: a prospective study of 10 patients and observations of enhanced sensory and motor function during stimulation. Neurosurgery 2005;56(2):290–7 [discussion: 290–7].
27. Monsalve GA. Motor cortex stimulation for facial chronic neuropathic pain: a review of the literature. Surg Neurol Int 2012;3(Suppl 4):S290–311.
28. Henderson JM, Boongird A, Rosenow JM, et al. Recovery of pain control by intensive reprogramming after loss of benefit from motor cortex stimulation for neuropathic pain. Stereotact Funct Neurosurg 2004;82(5–6):207–13.
29. Henderson JM, Lad SP. Motor cortex stimulation and neuropathic facial pain. Neurosurg Focus 2006; 21(6):E6.
30. Kanpolat Y, Savas A, Ugur HC, et al. The trigeminal tract and nucleus procedures in treatment of atypical facial pain. Surg Neurol 2005;64(Suppl 2): S96–100 [discussion: S100–1].
31. Mazars G, Merienne L, Cioloca C. [Treatment of certain types of pain with implantable thalamic stimulators]. Neurochirurgie 1974;20(2):117–24.
32. Coffey RJ. Deep brain stimulation for chronic pain: results of two multicenter trials and a structured review. Pain Med 2001;2(3):183–92.
33. Rasche D, Rinaldi PC, Young RF, Tronnier VM. Deep brain stimulation for the treatment of various chronic pain syndromes. Neurosurg Focus 2006;21(6):E8. Available at: http://dxdoiorg/103171/foc200621610.

Index

Note: Page numbers of article titles are in **boldface.**

Neurosurg Clin N Am 27 (2016) 371–374
http://dx.doi.org/10.1016/S1042-3680(16)30018-3
1042-3680/16/$ – see front matter

Printed and bound by CPI Group (UK) Ltd, Croydon, CR0 4YY

08/05/2025

01864686-0012